A Manual
of
Experimental Embryology

A Manual
of
Experimental Embryology

By

VIKTOR HAMBURGER

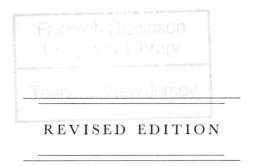
REVISED EDITION

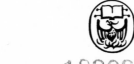
THE UNIVERSITY OF CHICAGO PRESS

CHICAGO & LONDON

Library of Congress Catalog Card Number: 60-14069

THE UNIVERSITY OF CHICAGO PRESS, CHICAGO 60637
The University of Chicago Press, Ltd., London W.C. 1

*© 1942, 1960 by The University of Chicago. Revised Edition
published 1960. Fourth Impression 1969. Printed in the
United States of America*

INTRODUCTION

Experimental embryology has achieved a prominent position in modern biology; its classical experiments and concepts are, by now, an integral part of biological thinking. Yet few students of biology have an opportunity to obtain a firsthand acquaintance with its methods and materials. This is due partly to the difficulties of providing the embryonic material and partly to the technical difficulties of experimentation on living embryos. However, a large number of classical experiments do not require exceptional manual skill and are suitable as "classroom" experiments. Most of the experiments described in the following pages have been made by advanced undergraduate and graduate students in a one-semester course which has been offered at Washington University since 1935. One of the main assets of such a course is to bring the student into intimate contact with the living, developing organism; and the enthusiastic response of the students indicates clearly the demand for such an approach to biology.

This *Manual* emphasizes the intrinsic factors of morphogenesis, that is, origin of form and of organs. It includes regeneration but gives little consideration to histogenesis and growth. In the selection of the experiments we were guided by practical considerations. Only those elementary experiments were chosen which do not require a high degree of manual skill[1] and which can be done in the limited time of a three-hour laboratory period. We excluded all experiments which require expensive apparatus, such as a micromanipulator. Special attention was paid to the development of simple and inexpensive instruments for operations. Only such living material as can be collected in the field or purchased at relatively small expense is recommended. All experiments were devised in such a way that sectioning of the material is not essential for the study of the results. For instance, regenerated lenses in amphibian larvae can be studied by making them opaque and thus visible by fixation in formaldehyde; chorio-allantoic grafts of limbs can be cleared and stained *in toto* with methylene blue; etc.

Another consideration which determined the selection of the experiments was their analytical value, that is, their expediency in illustrating important principles of morphogenesis. The theoretical significance of the experiments has been strongly emphasized. I believe that a course in an experimental branch of biology not only should acquaint the student with new facts but should strengthen

---

[1] In the Appendix the experiments are arranged in groups according to the technical difficulties involved.

v

his power of reasoning and his logical acuity as well. He should be aware of what an experiment proves and of what it does not prove. Each experiment or group of experiments is preceded by a brief outline of its theoretical implications. These general remarks integrate the different problems handled in the *Manual*, but they are not to be considered as a substitute for lectures or for textbooks. On the contrary, it is hoped that they will stimulate collateral reading. The bibliographies serve the same purpose. They are not complete but give references only to those articles which are directly related to the experiment under consideration and to pertinent review articles. A special chapter on gastrulation in amphibians was added, because familiarity with this phase of development is indispensable for experimental work on early embryos.

The experiments are organized according to a logical plan. This is not necessarily the sequence in which they should be taken up in the laboratory. The planning of the course work will depend largely on the availability of living material. To facilitate a flexible schedule, each experiment has been treated as a separate unit. The technical procedures are described for each experiment separately; they are not based on previous experience with other experiments. It is immaterial whether one starts with amphibians, with regeneration in planarians, or with chick experiments. The selection and arrangement of the exercises is left to the discretion of the instructor. A tentative schedule for a one-semester course will be found in the Appendix.

The instructions for technical manipulations are given in great detail. I hope that they will be useful not only for students but also for research workers in biology, experimental medicine, and related fields, who may find one or another of the techniques applicable to their own problems. The technical procedures have worked satisfactorily in our course, which does not mean that they cannot be further improved. I hope that the students will feel encouraged to develop their own initiative and resourcefulness in trying out new experiments and in improving the techniques and instruments.

The highly specialized technique of tissue culture has been omitted. The role of endocrines in morphogenesis is adequately presented in A. E. Adams' *Studies in Experimental Zoölogy* (1941), which contains all information necessary for experimentation in this field. Experiments on marine-animal eggs are dealt with in Just (1939).

I am indebted to many friends and colleagues. Many techniques described in the chapter on amphibians have been worked out in the laboratory of Dr. H. Spemann (Freiburg, Germany), with whom I was associated for many years. Dr. B. H. Willier and Dr. Mary Rawles generously made available their experiences with operations on the chick embryo. I am much obliged to Drs. L. G. Barth, G. Frankhauser, T. S. Hall, J. A. Moore, and C. Parmenter for personal communication of technical procedures. Grateful acknowledgment is made to all students and assistants who helped materially to improve the techniques and to revise the outlines. Dr. K. Gayer kindly read the manuscript and made many helpful suggestions.

I am grateful to Dr. R. G. Harrison for his kind permission to publish sketches of his unpublished stage series of *Ambystoma maculatum*. These sketches, as well as all other original drawings, were made by Miss S. E. Schweich. Acknowledgment is made to the Wistar Institute, Edwards Brothers, Incorporated, Akademische Verlags-Gesellschaft, and Springer-Verlag for permission to reproduce illustrations.

PREFACE TO THE SECOND EDITION

The revision of this *Manual* was undertaken in the belief that firsthand acquaintance with the methods of experimental morphogenesis, and direct contact with the living embryo, are still worthwhile objectives in the training of embryologists, despite the shift of emphasis in embryology to cellular and subcellular processes.

The aim of the book, as outlined in the Introduction to the first edition, as well as the general plan and the form of presentation of the material have remained unchanged. The book is not intended to be a handbook of experimental methods. It is organized within a conceptual framework, and methods and techniques, no matter how ingenious, are considered not as ends in themselves but subservient to problems and ideas. The practical aspects of the organization of the laboratory course are discussed in the enlarged Appendix.

Both the technical parts and the theoretical introductory remarks to the experiments have been thoroughly revised. Numerous technical advances and improvements of recent years have been incorporated. The directions for the execution of experiments have been made more specific, because the success of an experiment often depends on the strict observation of seemingly minor details. For the same reason, a set of basic rules for operations has been given (p. 41); it should be consulted by the student when he prepares and performs the experiments.

A few experiments have been omitted, and several important experiments have been added. The hormonal control of amphibian metamorphosis is illustrated by one simple but impressive experiment: the rearing of tadpoles in thyroxin solution. The method of rearing parts of early embryos in isolation (explantation), which has given valuable information on a number of significant problems and assumes increasing importance in conjunction with methods of cell dissociation and reaggregation, is represented by two simple experiments that are suitable as classroom experiments. They give an idea of the "self-differentiating" capacity of isolated parts but do not do justice to the versatility of this method. Advanced students might find it challenging to follow up this exercise with more subtle isolation, "sandwich," and dissociation experiments. The production of androgenetic haploid hybrids (according to directions kindly supplied by Dr. R. Briggs) was included because it focuses on several important problems concerning the role of the nucleus in development. This experiment and a few others are perhaps not suitable as classroom experiments, but they lend themselves to demonstrations by the instructor (see list of experi-

ix

ments, arranged according to the skill required to perform them, p. 204). The gradient theory is no longer handled in a separate part but is discussed in the part on regeneration, and several experiments pertinent to it are now included in this part.

This revision has profited greatly by the generous help and advice that I have received from many colleagues. Foremost among them is my friend, Dr. J. Holtfreter, of the University of Rochester, who let me share his unmatched knowledge of the ways of the amphibian embryo. Many of his valuable suggestions have been incorporated in this book, and many an error has been avoided, thanks to his vigilance. Dr. R. Briggs, of the University of Indiana, kindly made available his directions for the production of androgenetic haploid frog embryos. Dr. M. Steinberg, of the Carnegie Institute of Embryology, Baltimore, gave me advice on his culture medium; Dr. W. Muchmore, of the University of Rochester, advised me on isolation experiments and sterilization techniques; and Dr. V. Twitty, of Stanford University, gave advice on the handling of *Taricha*. Drs. W. Etkin, of the Albert Einstein College of Medicine, New York, and J. Kollros, of the State University of Iowa, kindly checked and improved the directions for the thyroxin experiment. Dr. Mary Rawles, of the Carnegie Institute of Embryology, Baltimore, very generously made available her wide experience in new and improved techniques of operating on the chick embryo, and Dr. W. Dossel, of the University of North Carolina Medical School, supplied me with information concerning the preparation of tungsten needles. I am most grateful to Dr. Dorothea Rudnick, of Albertus Magnus College, New Haven, for permission to reproduce her maps of the organ-forming areas of early chick embryos. Dr. E. Butler, of Princeton, placed at my disposal an unpublished modification of a technique for cartilage stain. Finally, I should like to express my gratitude to Miss Shirley Ross for her competent assistance in checking many of the experimental procedures and to Mrs. Bernadette Velick for the artistic execution of the new illustrations.

TABLE OF CONTENTS

xiii

LIST OF ILLUSTRATIONS

REFERENCE BOOKS ON EXPERIMENTAL EMBRYOLOGY
AND REGENERATION

BRACHET, J. 1950. Chemical embryology. New York: Interscience Publishers.

————. 1960. The biochemistry of development. New York: Pergamon Press.

CHILD, C. M. 1941. Patterns and problems of development. Chicago: University of Chicago Press.

DALCQ, A. M. 1938. Form and causality in early development. Cambridge, England: Cambridge University Press.

HUXLEY, J. S., and DE BEER, G. R. 1934. The elements of experimental embryology. Cambridge, England: Cambridge University Press.

KORSCHELT, E. 1927–31. Regeneration und Transplantation. 3 vols. Berlin: Borntraeger.

KÜHN, A. 1955. Vorlesungen über Entwicklungsphysiologie. Berlin: Springer.

LEHMANN, F. E. 1945. Einführung in die physiologische Embryologie. Basel: Birkhäuser.

MORGAN, T. H. 1927. Experimental embryology. New York: Columbia University Press.

NEEDHAM, A. E. 1952. Regeneration and wound healing. London: Methuen.

NEEDHAM, J. 1931. Chemical embryology. 3 vols. Cambridge, England: Cambridge University Press.

————. 1942. Biochemistry and morphogenesis. Cambridge, England: Cambridge University Press.

RAVEN, C. P. 1959. An outline of developmental physiology. New York: Pergamon Press.

SCHLEIP, W. 1929. Die Determination der Primitiventwicklung. Leipzig: Akademische Verlags-Gesellschaft.

SPEMANN, H. 1938. Embryonic development and induction. New Haven: Yale University Press.

WADDINGTON, C. H. 1956. Principles of embryology. New York: Macmillan Co.

WEISS, P. 1939. Principles of development. New York: Henry Holt & Co.

WILLIER, B. H., WEISS, P., and HAMBURGER, V. (eds.). 1955. Analysis of development. Philadelphia: W. B. Saunders Co.

The articles "Experimental embryology" and "Regeneration" in the *Encyclopaedia Britannica* by V. HAMBURGER give a brief outline of the major problems.

LABORATORY MANUALS OF EXPERIMENTAL EMBRYOLOGY

ADAMS, A. E. 1941. Studies in experimental zoölogy. 2d ed. Ann Arbor, Mich.: Edwards Bros., Inc.

COSTELLO, D. P., DAVIDSON, M. E., EGGERS, A., FOX, M. H., and HENLEY, C. 1957. Methods for obtaining and handling marine eggs and embryos. Marine Biological Laboratory, Woods Hole, Mass.

JUST, E. E. 1939. Basic methods for experiments on eggs of marine animals. Philadelphia: Blakiston & Sons Co.

RUGH, R. 1948. Experimental embryology: A manual of techniques and procedures. Minneapolis: Burgess Publishing Co.

PART I
EQUIPMENT AND INSTRUMENTS

A. OPTICAL OUTFIT

A low-power binocular microscope is indispensable for experimental embryological and regeneration studies. Any standard model is acceptable. The V-base with substage mirror is not necessary for most experiments; on the contrary, it is preferable to have the glass stage for the operation dish directly on the work table so that the arms of the operator have optimal support. Magnifications ranging between ×6 and ×24 are sufficient for most purposes. For illumination, any lamp that is mounted on an adjustable support, that has a strong light source, and that gives an evenly illuminated field may be used. Precautions must be taken against heating of the operation dish. In our laboratory, makeshift lamps are in use; these consist of a 75-watt bulb, mounted inside a tin can, and a 500-cc. Pyrex boiling flask filled with water, which serves as a condenser and cooler; both items are clamped on an ordinary iron support. A Beebe binocular magnifying glass, which is worn like a pair of spectacles, has been found to be very useful on many occasions, for instance, in preparing glass needles, in selecting amphibian embryos, or in hypophysectomy of frogs.

B. GLASS INSTRUMENTS
(Use soft glass for all instruments; do not use Pyrex)

Material
    glass tubing, 6–7 mm. in outer diameter
    glass tubing 9–10 mm. in outer diameter
    glass rod 5–6 mm. in outer diameter
    rubber tubing 11–12 mm. in outer diameter
    rubber tubing 8–9 mm. in outer diameter
    rubber caps for pipettes
    cover glass
    Bunsen burner
    iron support
    file
    diamond pencil[1]

1. *Pipettes.*—Use both 6–7-mm. and 9–10-mm. glass tubing. Cut pieces of about 8 inches (for 2 pipettes). Heat the middle of the piece over the Bunsen burner; roll the piece constantly between your fingers to avoid one-sided melt-

---

[1] In using the diamond pencil, scratch only halfway around the rod or tube and then break the pieces apart by gentle pressure. Do not mark around the entire circumference.

ing. When the glass is softened, pull slowly, holding your hands horizontally until the desired diameter is reached. Wide-mouthed and gradually tapering pipettes may best be made over a burner with wing top, which gives a broad flame. Cut the pipettes to the desired length with the diamond pencil. Hold both openings in the flame to smooth the edges. Fit rubber caps over the wide end. Prepare pipettes of different widths ranging between 2 and 5 mm. Prepare several of each kind.

2. *Capillary pipettes.*—Prepare a pipette with a narrow lumen and short neck, as under paragraph 1, above. In a second step, hold the narrow part near the neck over the low or medium-size flame of the Bunsen burner and pull again (Fig. 1, *m, lower arrow*). Cut the pipette to size by scratching one side with the diamond pencil. If you find it difficult to obtain straight capillary pipettes by this technique, use the following trick: Prepare a short-neck pipette with narrow lumen, as before. Cut it off a considerable distance from the tapering region and bend the narrow end into a hook by holding it in the flame. Hook the pipette over a ring on an iron support placed near the edge of the table, with the pipette suspended over the edge so that it will not drop on the table when heated (Fig. 1, *n*). Heat an area near the tapering part very gently and cautiously with a low Bunsen-burner flame or a microburner. When properly heated, the tube will be drawn out into a very fine capillary tube of almost microscopic dimension by the weight of the lower, wide part. If too much heat is applied, the tube will be pulled apart and drop. Even so, it can be saved by placing a container, laid out with cotton, at some distance directly under the suspended pipette. Cut off the fine end with a diamond pencil.

3. *Microburner.*—The microburner is a small gas burner used for the preparation of very fine glass needles and other instruments. It is best made of an ordinary injection needle, whose pointed end is cut off and whose wide end is fastened in rubber tubing connecting with the gas jet (Fig. 1, *b*). It is mounted in a horizontal position by clamping it on a support, or otherwise. The optimal length of the flame is 5 mm. or less. The size of the flame may be controlled by a clamp on the rubber tubing or directly by the gas jet.

Microburners of glass may be easily made of 6–7-mm. tubing. Prepare a capillary tube according to section 2 and cut off the narrowest part with the diamond pencil (Fig. 1, *m, upper arrow*). If the opening is too small, the flame will seal it off by melting the edge. The flame must be of blue color; a yellow flame indicates the melting of the edge. Control the gas supply with a clamp.

4. *Micropipette (after Spemann).*—This capillary pipette (Fig. 1, *l*) with a lateral hole was used by Spemann in the original transplantation experiments on gastrulae (1918), in conjunction with a fine steel knife. Most transplantations are now done with glass needles (see below), but the Spemann pipette is still useful in picking up and transferring small transplants and explants. It is prepared in the following way: Pull out a fine pipette, about 1–2 mm. in nar-

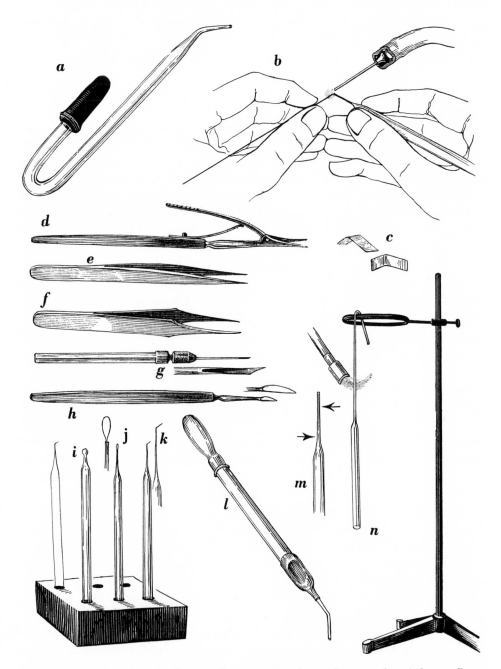

FIG. 1.—Instruments for operating on embryos. *a*, micropipette; *b*, preparation of glass needle on the microburner; *c*, glass bridges; *d*, iridectomy scissors; *e*, *f*, watchmaker forceps; *g*, fine steel knife, prepared by sharpening of sewing needle; *h*, Knapp iris needle; *i*, glass rod with ball tip; *j*, hair loop; *k*, glass needle; *l*, Spemann micropipette; *m*, *n*, preparation of capillary pipette (see text).

rowest diameter, using 7–8-mm. glass tubing. Make the handle at least 10–12 cm. long. To blow a hole in the handle, proceed as follows: Seal the capillary end of the pipette by holding it in the flame. Attach a piece of rubber tubing to the wide end of the pipette. Bring one side of the wall of the handle, near the point where it tapers, very near the flame of a Bunsen burner and heat it thoroughly until it is soft. Take it out of the flame and, while it is hot, blow air through the rubber tubing. The air cannot escape through the sealed capillary and will blow out the soft glass in the form of a large, sausage-shaped, thin-walled bubble. The bubble usually explodes instantly, or it can be easily removed. Scratch the circumference of the hole with a diamond pencil and break off carefully all glass particles up to this mark. Smooth the edge of the hole over the flame. Cut off the closed capillary; be sure to make a straight cut. It is convenient to have the capillary opening slightly bent. Hold it horizontally over the flame of the microburner in such a way that the hole faces you and the capillary end points to your left. Gently heat the lower wall of the capillary near its opening. The end piece will then bend by its own weight. With a forceps bend it farther, until it is at an angle of about 120° to the straight part. Next cover the hole with a rubber membrane. Cut a piece of rubber-latex tubing to cover the lateral hole, moisten the pipette and rubber piece, and slip the latter over the hole. It must fit very tightly. Fit a rubber cap over the wide end. The lateral hole can also be prepared on a rotating grindstone.

Use of the micropipette.—Place your right thumb on the rubber membrane over the hole. Draw in water, using the distal cap, until the narrow end is filled almost to the level of the hole. While the opening is under water, squirt out a small amount of water by gentle pressure on the membrane over the hole. Retain the pressure and, under the binocular microscope, place the opening of the pipette over the object. Then release the pressure slowly. The object will be drawn into the capillary portion and can be transferred. A slight pressure on the membrane suffices to release it again.

A simplified model of a micropipette is illustrated in Figure 1, *a*.[2]

A good micropipette must hold water in the capillary end, that is, no water must drip out when it is held with the narrow opening pointing downward.

5. *Glass needles (Fig. 1, k)*.—These needles are the universal cutting instruments for extirpation and transplantation experiments on amphibian and chick embryos. They consist of a handle with a short, rapidly tapering neck and with a short, pointed needle attached to its end at an angle of approximately 120° (Fig. 1, *k*). The student should practice the preparing of glass needles before he starts operations. Different techniques of preparing them are in use; they are adapted to the skill and the temperament of the experimenter. First prepare from 6 to 8 handles, using a glass rod 5–6 mm. in diameter. Hold the middle of the piece in the flame of a Bunsen burner in a horizontal position and

2 This sketch was kindly supplied by Dr. Mary Rawles.

6

pull the ends apart rapidly as soon as the middle part is very soft. Break the thin connecting thread apart and pull out each thread in a second step by heating it close to the neck over a Bunsen or preferably a microburner. The handle should now be straight, tapering to a very fine, elastic thread, much thinner than a hair. Break off the thread where it gets very fine and use the broken-off piece or scraps of fine thread for the final step, the pulling of the needle proper. Hold a piece of this thread between the thumb and finger of your left hand and hold the handle in your right hand. Bring the fine tips of thread and handle to contact, at an angle of 120°. Put the free fingers against one another to get better control (Fig. 1, b). In this position, move the contact point slowly toward the flame of the microburner. At the moment that the contact point heats up and the two threads fuse, pull them apart. Some people pull slowly; others accomplish this better in a rapid, jerky motion. The thread will be spun out to an exceedingly fine fiber. The needle must now be cut to the appropriate length. This is done by clipping with a fine watchmaker forceps under the binocular dissecting scope. The needle should have a pointed end and should not be elastic at the tip. It is not possible to give detailed instructions as to thickness and length of the needle, since this depends on the consistency of the embryonic material, which differs with the stage of development and also with respect to the part to be cut. It is advisable to prepare needles of different thicknesses and lengths and try them out on the embryo. Consult the laboratory instructor if you have difficulty in using the needle.

In a simplified technique of preparing the needles, the end points of the two finely drawn-out handles are brought in contact at an angle of 120°, moved slowly toward the low flame of a Bunsen burner or a microburner, and pulled apart at the moment when they fuse. In this way, two needles are obtained at once. A Beebe binocular magnifier is of great service in preparing needles.

Prepare 6–8 needles in advance in order to have a supply on hand in case one breaks during an operation. Some investigators use fine Tungsten needles instead of glass needles (see p. 10).

6. *Hair loop (Spemann) and platinum wire loop (Fig. 1, j).*—Loops are used for handling living embryos or transplants. Spemann found the very fine, soft, and elastic hair of babies particularly suitable for this purpose. The hair of adults is too coarse. The hair is mounted in a handle in the following way. Prepare a number of fine capillary tubes as in section 2. Cut off with a diamond pencil near the tapering part at a point where the lumen is just wide enough to hold the two ends of the hair. Cut pieces of hair about 3 cm. long and maneuver the ends of the hair into the capillary opening, as follows: Hold the handle in your left hand, and with your right hand pick up a piece of hair with a watchmaker forceps. Under the binocular dissecting scope, work first one end of the hair and then the other into the capillary opening and adjust the size of

the loop to a diameter of about 3–4 mm. Avoid breaking or crushing the hair. To seal the hair into the capillary, melt a small piece of paraffin on a glass plate (slide) and dip the hair loop into it. A small amount of liquid paraffin will be sucked into the end of the tube by capillary force and will harden instantly. Sometimes a film of paraffin will remain in the hair loop. To remove it, warm a piece of filter paper on a slide and touch the hair to the warm paper; avoid melting the paraffin in the handle. Prepare a stock of hair loops of different sizes.

The hair loop has one disadvantage: it cannot be sterilized in heat because this melts the paraffin. For this reason, loops of platinum wire are used in some laboratories. They can be mounted in the same way as hair loops.

7. *Glass rods with ball tips.*—These rods (Fig. 1, *i*) are used to imprint grooves in the agar or wax bottom of operation dishes, to hold the embryos. Cut a piece of glass rod (5–6 mm. in diam.) long enough for 2 handles. Heat in the middle and pull out to a moderately thin rod. Break off the slender part near the neck and hold the tip of the handle in a vertical position in the flame of a microburner with the tip pointing downward. It will melt and form a ball. The neck connecting the ball with the handle should be short and wide; otherwise the ball will break off.

8. *Glass bridges.*—Glass bridges (Fig. 1, *c*) are used in transplantations of amphibian embryos to hold the transplant in position until it is healed in. Using diamond pencil and ruler, cut a cover glass (thickness No. 2) into small strips, 3–4 mm. wide. Cut each strip into small rectangular pieces, 10–12 mm. long. Take up each piece with a watchmaker forceps and pull its four edges slowly through the microburner until all sharp and rough projections disappear. All edges must be absolutely smooth. Grasp each glass piece on one narrow end and hold it in a slanted position over the microburner in such a way that an area a short distance from the other end is heated from below. The end opposite the forceps will then bend down by its own weight. The glass bridge, when finished, must stand firmly on its narrow edges.

The size and angle of the glass bridge must be adapted to the material. The bridge can be easily cleaned and sterilized by pulling it quickly through a Bunsen or alcohol burner. Prepare 6–8 bridges of slightly different angles and lengths. Keep them in a covered dish.

9. *Holders for glass instruments.*—Each student should have a wooden holder for glass needles, hair loops, etc. The holder is prepared from a piece of solid wood, about $20 \times 7 \times 3$ cm., with 2 rows of holes slightly wider than the diameters of the handles and bored at a distance of about 3 cm. from each other (Fig. 1, *lower left*). Pipettes are kept on a pipette support made of 2 connected rows of undulating heavy steel wire, the back row being somewhat higher than the front row.

C. METAL INSTRUMENTS

1. *Scalpels, scissors, and forceps.*—Scalpels, scissors, and forceps of different sizes will be needed for many manipulations. Stainless-steel instruments are preferable. Chromium-plated instruments are not recommended because particles of the plating are likely to chip off when one tries to resharpen the instruments.

2. *Watchmaker forceps.*—These forceps (Fig. 1, *e, f*) are universal tools and indispensable for work on embryos. They must have very fine points and must work very smoothly, that is, they must respond to the slightest pressure. Instruments made of high-grade steel (stainless, if possible) should be selected. Two types of such forceps are on the market—one with gradually tapering ends and one with shoulders. The latter usually have finer points. Watchmaker forceps may be purchased from laboratory supply houses or from wholesale watchmakers' or jewelers' tool companies.

Even the best watchmaker forceps usually require further sharpening before use. This is done on a fine-grain oilstone under the binocular dissecting scope. Place a drop of oil on the stone. Bring the points in contact with each other and set them sidewise on the oil stone. Gently press the points down with the tips of the index finger and stroke them without exerting much pressure. Continue this on both sides until very fine sharp points are achieved. Finish the polishing by gently rotating each point individually on the stone, and then both together. It is essential that the points fit exactly together. Clean the forceps carefully and remove all traces of oil before using them. The forceps require frequent resharpening. Rust can be removed with scouring powder.

3. *Iridectomy scissors.*—These scissors are the finest on the market. They, as well as the finest lancets, have been taken over by the experimental embryologist from the ophthalmologist. Some investigators use the scissors for operations on chick and amphibian embryos; for instance, Dr. Harrison did many of his experiments on amphibian tail-bud stages with this instrument. Iridectomy scissors are too expensive for class use, and all operations described in this *Manual* were devised for the glass-needle technique. However, they are the instrument of choice for the amputation of limbs and tails in amphibian regeneration experiments (p. 192), and it is suggested that several of them be available, to be used jointly by the class for these operations.

Several models of iridectomy scissors are on the market; they are equally useful for our purpose. In some types (DeWecker, McClure) the blades are closed by pressure on both handles (spring handles); in another type, one blade is fixed on the handle and the other, shorter blade is movable (Fig. 1, *d*).

4. *Steel knives and lancets.*—Very fine, sharp, and pointed steel knives are indispensable for delicate operations, particularly on the chick embryo. The finest knives on the market are iris and cataract knives. Many different models

9

are available. We have found the single-edged straight Knapp iris needle with a half-spear point (Fig. 1, *h*), or similar types, particularly useful.

Students should learn to prepare their own very fine all-purpose knives by sharpening sewing or beading needles. The material must be of the very best quality, otherwise no sharp edges and points can be obtained. We prefer fine sewing or embroidery needles made in England (Milwards, Harpers, etc.). It takes some practice to sharpen the needle properly (Fig. 1, *g*). Place a drop of oil on a fine-grain oil stone. Hold the needle between the fingers or mount it in a metal holder with screw chuck. Flatten the point in two planes which meet at an acute angle in a sharp edge. It is essential to have a very sharp end point. For use, mount the knife in a metal holder. The knives have to be resharpened frequently.

5. *Tungsten needles.*—The following directions have been kindly supplied by Dr. W. E. Dossel. They are a combination of the two techniques described by him in *Laboratory Investigation,* 7:171, 1958. These needles have several advantages over glass needles: they are unbreakable; they are opaque and therefore clearly visible during the operation; they can be sterilized by pulling them through the flame; and they can be given any shape.

Use tungsten wire of a diameter of between 0.005 and 0.01 in. Cut it in pieces 1 inch long and seal each piece in a handle prepared from Pyrex glass tubing (3-mm. outside diameter) that has been drawn out into a short capillary tube; its opening should be just wide enough to hold the wire. The wire should be straight and protrude about half its length. Seal it by melting the glass around it

The preparation of the sharp point is done in two steps.

a) Place the tip of the wire in an oxygen-gas flame just above the bright inner cone. The wire will glow white and then abruptly begin to disappear at the tip, at which time it should be quickly removed from the flame. Heat the tip only.

b) For the second step use a bath of fused sodium nitrite. Support a porcelain or, preferably, fire-clay crucible on a triangle, fill it to the depth of $\frac{1}{2}$ inch with anhydrous sodium nitrite, and heat it with an air-gas or oxygen-gas blast burner until the chemical is fused. The wire is sharpened by dipping it into and withdrawing it from the molten chemical. The rapidity with which the process proceeds is dependent upon the temperature of the bath; a higher temperature (indicated by the appearance of an excessively yellowish glow) removes the metal more rapidly but produces a somewhat uneven, pitted surface, while a temperature that is too low (suggested by the formation of a crust about the periphery of the bath) leads to the formation of a bead about the wire that effectively insulates it from the action of the chemical. When the temperature is properly adjusted, the metal is removed at a moderate rate, leaving the surface of the developing needle smooth, bright, and free from oxidation. The shape of the point can be varied at will, from a long, very sharp point to a sharply tapering, somewhat blunted point, by controlling the depth of immersion and the frequency of immersion and withdrawal. Obviously, care must be taken not to damage the point by touching it to the bottom of the crucible. After the needle is completed to satisfaction, a crust of varicolored crystalline matter will be found to adhere to the shank, but this may be easily removed by washing the entire needle in very hot water for a few minutes.

There is some inherent danger associated with this latter technic. The fused chemical is exceedingly corrosive and will pit not only porcelain but also fused quartz, vycor glass, and even fire clay to some extent. It is best, therefore, to discard the porcelain crucible when pitting is dangerously deep and to use thick fire-clay crucibles when a temperature source can be had that is sufficiently hot to maintain the bath in a fused condition. Further, protective glasses should be worn in the event the crucible should break. During the dipping process, hold the handle of the wire with asbestos gloves.

D. GLASS DISHES FOR OPERATIONS AND FOR RAISING OF OPERATED ANIMALS

Crystallizing dishes and large ($7\frac{1}{2}$-in.) finger-bowl dishes are used for keeping jelly masses of amphibian eggs, planarians, etc.

Petri dishes, finger-bowl dishes of ordinary size ($4\frac{1}{2}$ in.), or Syracuse watch glasses are used for keeping small numbers of eggs and individual specimens. They will be needed for many purposes and should be available in large quantities. Each student should be given several Petri dishes, several finger bowls, and from 6 to 12 Syracuse dishes.

Section dishes ($2\frac{1}{4}$ in.) are very practical but expensive.

Lids (cut to size out of ordinary window glass) should be provided for every dish.

Operation dishes for amphibian embryos.—Syracuse dishes may be used, but they are rather shallow. Furniture-caster dishes are best suited for our purpose. Since naked embryos in concentrated Holtfreter solution tend to stick to the glass surface, it is necessary to cover the bottom with a suitable surface material. Agar is most widely used and strongly recommended. It can be readily sterilized, it has the right consistency, and grooves for holding the embryo during operations can be cut with a sturdy glass needle or a small knife.

Prepare a 2 or 3 per cent agar solution in concentrated Holtfreter solution and pour it in the caster dishes or other operation and culture dishes. The layer should be just thick enough to allow the digging of grooves to hold an embryo. If the layer is too thick, the volume of culture medium is cut down too much. Cover the dish with a sterile lid and be sure to keep it covered. For some operations (e.g., vital staining of gastrulae) a harder substrate is preferable,

11

and beeswax or a mixture of beeswax and paraffin (50° melting point) is recommended. The surface can be sterilized by touching it with the flame of a Bunsen burner. Grooves to hold the embryo during operation can be impressed with a cold ball tip in the warm wax. Paraffin and wax bottoms sometimes get loose and float on the surface. To prevent this, use the following procedure. Cut three or four pieces of glass rod, somewhat shorter than the diameter of the dish; dip them into liquid wax and place them on the bottom of the dish while they are still warm, so that they will stick to the bottom. Then pour the liquid wax into the dish.

Dishes for rearing of embryos.—The delicate, young stages, up to early tail-bud stages, are best kept in Syracuse dishes or furniture-caster dishes with agar bottom, as described in the preceding paragraph. For older embryos and swimming larvae we recommend paraffined paper cups of the type used for jellies or ice cream (Lily cups and other brands). They are much less expensive than glassware and can be obtained in quantity in a number of different sizes. Adequate sizes are: for embryos, 2-ounce dishes with an upper diameter of about 2 inches, and for swimming larvae about 4-ounce dishes with an upper diameter of 3 inches. All paper cups must be coated with paraffin. Some brands can be obtained with a paraffin coat; all others have to be dipped in liquid paraffin. All dishes should be covered. It is best to use square glass plates cut to size. They, as well as the dishes, have to be sterilized before they are used.

E. STERILIZATION OF INSTRUMENTS

Sterilization of all glassware, instruments, culture media, towels, etc. is imperative for all work on chick and early amphibian embryos. A vertical or horizontal autoclave or water-bath sterilizer can be used for dishes, pipettes, towels (all wrapped in paper towels), and flasks with culture media. Watch-maker forceps, knives, needles, scissors, and other metal instruments must be thoroughly cleaned before use. They are best kept in 70 per cent alcohol during the operations, in a jar with cotton at its bottom, and pulled through the flame before use. Carefully avoid bringing the embryo in contact with alcohol. Glass needles and hair loops are too delicate to be autoclaved without elaborate precautions. To keep them clean, dip them in 70 per cent alcohol and then in sterile culture medium before use. As the best protection against infection, it is recommended that the needles be discarded after they have been used for one set of operations and that new needles be prepared shortly before use.

PART II
EXPERIMENTS ON AMPHIBIAN EMBRYOS

A. BACKGROUND MATERIAL AND PRELIMINARIES TO EXPERIMENTAL WORK

1. LIVING MATERIAL

a) AMPHIBIANS COMMONLY USED FOR EXPERIMENTAL WORK, AND THEIR BREEDING HABITS

The following brief survey is limited to the few North American forms that, because of their relative abundance and wide geographic distribution, are most commonly used for experimental work. Other, more rare, forms that may be abundant locally would probably serve many experimental purposes as well. However, one cannot take it for granted that two closely related forms will always give the same experimental results. The differences between related anurans with respect to lens induction (p. 114) and between different urodeles with respect to Wolffian lens regeneration (p. 197) may serve as a warning. Furthermore, some species lend themselves for operations better than others because of their consistency, viability, or other properties. To avoid experimental failures caused by choice of unsuitable material, we have indicated for each experiment the species that are recommended. Those listed are the forms used either by the original investigator or in our classroom experiments.

Most of the data presented below are taken from the excellent amphibian handbooks of Bishop (1943), Stebbins (1953), and Wright and Wright (1949). These three books contain a wealth of information on all North American *Amphibia,* including maps of their geographic distribution, keys for identification, and extensive bibliographies. The last-mentioned work contains well illustrated keys for anuran eggs and tadpoles, including extensive data on egg size, egg color, egg membranes, and shape and size of egg clusters (see also Orton, 1952). Corresponding data for urodeles may be found in Bishop (1941). For information on eggs and larvae of the California urodeles see Twitty (1936, 1942). A key for European anuran tadpoles, including data on egg clusters, may be found in Kopsch (1952). For questions concerning taxonomy see Schmidt (1953) and Riemer (1958; *Taricha*).

Students who are interested in getting more information on general biological aspects and behavior of their experimental animals are referred to Noble (1931) and Oliver (1955). A field guide by Conant (1958) is available in the Petersen series.

ORDER *Urodela*

FAMILY AMBYSTOMIDAE

1. *Ambystoma*[1] *maculatum* Shaw, frequently referred to as *A. punctatum*. Spotted salamander. Average size, 170 mm. Color, deep bluish-black, with two rows of rounded yellow or orange spots on the back. Ventral side lighter. The most common *Ambystoma*. Widely used for experiments.

Breeding places: Woodland ponds and slowly running streams.

Breeding season: Varies considerably with latitude, from February in southern regions, March in central midwest, to April and May in northern regions. The breeding season in a given locality lasts for several weeks. The animals spend the rest of the year in burrows or under stones and logs on land.

Egg masses: 100–150 eggs, each in its own jelly membrane, are held together in a common jelly envelope, which is firm and globular in shape and clear or milky. They are attached to sticks or float freely within 8–10 inches from the surface. Egg diameter, $2\frac{1}{2}$–3 mm.

Range: Nova Scotia, w. to Wisconsin and s. to Georgia and Texas (Bishop, 1943).

2. *Ambystoma tigrinum* Green. Tiger salamander. This is the largest native *Ambystoma,* averaging 200 mm. Deep-brown to black on dorsal side, olive-yellow on ventral side. Markings dorsally and laterally are irreguar olive-brown to brownish-yellow blotches, much duller and more irregular than in *A. maculatum.*

Breeding places: Permanent or temporary ponds.

Breeding season: In all regions slightly earlier than *A. maculatum* (January–March). During the rest of the year the animals are on land, hidden under stones, logs, etc.

Egg masses: Average, 30–50 eggs; their common jelly envelope is softer, less firm, than in *A. maculatum.* They are usually fastened to twigs and branches 12 inches or more under the surface. Egg diameter, 3 mm.

Range: From Long Island s. to n. Florida, w. to Texas and Arkansas, and n. to Minnesota and Ontario (Bishop, 1943).

3. *Ambystoma opacum* Gravenhorst. Marbled salamander. The smallest of the three, about 100 mm. Color, black, with light markings on the back and on the sides. Their color is dull gray in the ♀ and bright in the ♂, very variable in size and shape.

Breeding places: This form does not lay its eggs in the water but hides them in shallow grooves, under leaves, or under logs in woods. The breeding places are on the margin of temporary ponds or swampy places that are dry at the

---

[1] The spelling "Ambystoma" has been adopted in this *Manual,* following the rules of nomenclature. Most experimental embryologists use the traditional spelling "Amblystoma." There can be no doubt that the latter is linguistically correct, meaning "blunted mouth," whereas the one which enjoys priority is meaningless and probably a typographical error. (See Dr. Harrison's remarks in Jour. Exper. Zool., **41**:351 n.)

16

breeding season but that will be submerged later in the year. Many females migrate to the same place, so that one can usually collect from many nests in the same location.

Breeding season: September and October.

Egg masses: The eggs are laid singly, not held together by a common envelope. Particles usually stick to the surface of the eggs, whereby the eggs are well concealed. The membranes will swell, and the larvae will hatch when the eggs are placed in water. Egg diameter, 2.7 mm.

Range: From New Hampshire to Florida, w. to Louisiana and Texas, Mississippi Basin, n. to Arkansas, Missouri, Indiana, and Wisconsin (Bishop, 1943).

FAMILY SALAMANDRIDAE

4. *Diemictylus viridescens* (=*Triturus viridescens*). Common spotted newt. Average size, 85 mm. Color in the aquatic form: dorsal side, olive-green; ventral side, light to bright yellow. Small black spots scattered over both sides. A series of black spots on either side of the dorsal mid-line. The land form, called "eft," is bright red. During the breeding season the males can be easily recognized by their broad, wavy tail fins and by the presence of black bars on the ventral surface of the hind legs.

Breeding places: Ponds, lakes, and slowly moving waters.

Breeding season: Variable with latitude. April to June and more extended than in frogs and *Ambystoma.*

Eggs are deposited singly on leaves of *Vallisneria, Elodea,* and other aquatic plants. The female grasps a leaf with her hind legs, deposits the egg on it, and then folds the leaf so that the egg is almost entirely concealed. The outermost egg capsule is sticky, milky white. Egg diameter, 1.5 mm.

Females will lay eggs readily in the laboratory. They should be kept in large aquaria, and plenty of fresh *Elodea* or *Vallisneria* or narrow slips of paper should be provided. To insure fertilization, a number of males should be added. They will court and clasp the females and deposit their spermatophores in the aquarium

Range: Ontario, e. and s. states, w. to Texas, Kansas, Missouri, n. to Minnesota.

5. *Taricha torosa* Rathke (=*Triturus torosus*). California newt. Average size, 170 mm. Different shades of brown on the upper side, orange or yellow on the ventral side.

Breeding places: Streams, ponds, and reservoirs.

Breeding season: Varies with altitude. January and February in low altitudes; until early summer in high altitudes.

Egg masses: 10–25 eggs form a firm, globular cluster. They are attached to water plants. Egg diameter, 2–2.8 mm.

17

Range: Along the California coast; a subspecies, *T. sierrae,* on the western slopes of the Sierra. Twitty has described two other California species, *T. granulosa* and *T. rivularis,* which have been used by him for hybridization experiments. For description and distribution see Twitty (1936, 1942) and Riemer (1958).

ORDER *Anura*

FAMILY RANIDAE

6. *Rana pipiens* Schreber. Leopard frog. Average length, 80–90 mm. Dorsal side with rounded or oval dark spots, rather irregularly spaced. Smaller spots on the sides. Ventral side, whitish or yellowish. The males can be easily recognized by the swelling at the thumbs. The commonest and most widely used frog.

Breeding places: In ponds and swampy marshlands.

Breeding season: Early spring (March and April). The adults spend the summer on land and hibernate in the water, hidden beneath stones or logs.

Egg masses: Contain approximately 3,000 eggs. The jelly membranes of the individual eggs stick together, but they are not inclosed in a common envelope. They are laid near the surface; usually a considerable number of masses are deposited at the same place. Egg diameter, 1.7 mm.

Range: Most parts of the United States except the Pacific Coast.

7. *Rana palustris* LeConte. The pickerel frog. Average size, 70 mm., smaller than *Rana pipiens.* Upper side, pale brownish with dark spots; these are larger and more regularly arranged than those of *R. pipiens,* namely, in two distinct rows. They are oblong or square. Underside, yellowish-white. *R. palustris* can be easily distinguished from *R. pipiens* by the bright-yellow color of the underside of the thighs. Males have thickened thumbs.

Breeding places: Cold springs and streams, ravines, ponds.

Breeding season: Late April and May. The adults spend the summer in marshy places, ravines, moss bogs, etc., and hibernate in water covered by logs and stones.

Egg masses: Contain about 2,000 eggs. They are laid in shallow water and are usually attached to sticks. The masses are much like those of *R. pipiens,* but the eggs can be easily recognized by the brown animal pole and the yellow vegetal pole, in contrast to the black and white of *R. pipiens.* Egg diameter, 1.8 mm.

Range: N. to Canada, w. to Great Plains, s. to Louisiana and Florida.

8. *Rana sylvatica* LeConte. Wood frog. The smallest of the common frogs, 65 mm. Upper side, gray to brownish with dark streaks on both sides of the head and a few scattered dark spots. Lower side, whitish. Males have swollen thumbs.

Breeding places: Still waters, ponds, transient pools in woods.

Breeding season: Slightly earlier than the other common frogs, middle of March to April, as soon as the ice has melted. The frogs spend the summer in the woods and hibernate on land, in woods, under cover.

Egg masses: Contain about 2,000 eggs. They are similar to those of *R. pipiens* but more globular, and individual eggs are less crowded, i.e., outer jelly membranes are thicker. Most frequently attached to water plants, twigs, etc. Egg diameter, 1.9 mm.

Range: N. to Maine, s. to North Carolina, w. to Missouri.

9. *Rana catesbeiana* Shaw. Bullfrog. The largest of all native frogs; up to 17–20 cm. Upper side, brown; ventral side, white. Males have thickened thumbs.

Breeding places: Lakes, ponds, brooks, marshy swamps, streams. The adults stay in the water throughout the year. The tadpoles spend two years in the larval stage.

Breeding season: Later than most other frogs: June and July in northern parts, somewhat earlier in southern parts.

Egg masses: Contain more eggs than those of other frogs, 10,000 and more being reported. They are laid as a surface film. The jelly is loose and gelatinous and less compact than that of the other common frogs. The egg masses are deposited among brush at the edge of the ponds. Egg diameter, 1.3 mm.

Range: Eastern states to the Rocky Mountains.

BIBLIOGRAPHY

BISHOP, S. C. 1941. The salamanders of New York. New York State Mus. Bull. 324. Albany: University of the State of New York.
———. 1943. Handbook of salamanders. Ithaca, N.Y.: Comstock Pub. Co.
CONANT, ROGER. 1958. A field guide to reptiles and amphibians of eastern North America. Boston: Houghton Mifflin.
KOPSCH, FR. 1952. Die Entwicklung des braunen Grasfrosches, *Rana Fusca* Roesel. Stuttgart: Georg Thieme Verlag.
NOBLE, G. KINGSLEY. 1931. The biology of *Amphibia*. New York: McGraw-Hill.
OLIVER, J. A. 1955. Natural history of North America amphibians and reptiles. New York: Van Nostrand.
ORTON, G. 1952. Key to the genera of tadpoles in the United States and Canada. Amer. Midland Naturalist, **47:**382–95.
RIEMER, W. J. 1958. Variation and systematic relationships within the salamander genus *Taricha*. Univ. Calif. Pub. Zoöl., **56:**301–90.
SCHMIDT, K. P. 1953. A check list of North American amphibians and reptiles. American Society of Ichthyology and Herpetology. Chicago: University of Chicago Press.
STEBBINS, R. C. 1951. Amphibians of western North America. Berkeley: University of California Press.
———. 1954. Amphibians of western North America. New York: McGraw-Hill.
TWITTY, V. C. 1936. Correlated genetic and embryological experiments on *Triturus*. I. Hybridization: Development of three species of *Triturus* and their hybrid combinations. II. Transplantation: The embryological basis of species differences in pigment pattern. Jour. Exper. Zool., **74:**239–302.

———. 1942. The species of California *Triturus*. Copeia, No. 2, p. 65.

WRIGHT, A. H., and WRIGHT, A. A. 1949. Handbook of frogs and toads of the United States and Canada. Ithaca, N.Y.: Comstock Pub. Co.

b) STAGE SERIES, RATES OF DEVELOPMENT, TEMPERATURE TOLERANCE, AND OTHER DATA

For practical purposes it is desirable to break up the continuous process of development into discrete "stages" and to agree on standardized "stage series" for convenient reference in descriptive and experimental work. The stages should be characterized by easily identifiable external features. In cold-blooded animals stage seriations in terms of age are useless because the rate of development varies with temperature. It should be understood that in the stage series listed below the time intervals between any two successive stages are not constant but differ from stage to stage. The series for different forms have been worked out by different authors and their initials will be added to the stage numbers. This practice will be followed throughout this *Manual*.

ORDER *Urodela*

1. *Ambystoma maculatum*.—Harrison's excellent series for this widely used salamander is the most complete and most perfect stage series devised so far; it has been used as a model for other urodele series. It is not published, but it is widely circulated through the courtesy of the author and generally adopted by experimental embryologists. It covers with 46 stages the period from the uncleaved egg to the stage in which the larva begins to feed. The stages are depicted in Figure 45.

Rate of development.—This rate varies with temperature and other external factors.[2] Table 1 is compiled for practical purposes. The data are combined from Dempster (1933), J. Moore (1939), and my own notes, all three of which are in close agreement.

OTHER DATA ON NORMAL DEVELOPMENT

Rupture of vitelline membrane: Late neurula stage.

First movements: Stages H32–H34 (for details see p. 136).

First heartbeat: H34.

Hatching: H40–H42 = 15–19 days.

Beginning of feeding: H45–H46 = 25 days.

Metamorphosis: Varies considerably with feeding, etc.: from 70 days (at maximal feeding; Twitty and Schwind, 1931) to 120 days or more.

---

[2] DuShane and Hutchinson (1941, p. 247) indicate that in all probability genetic differences in developmental rates exist between eastern and middle-western races.

Growth curves: May be found in Harrison (1929), Stone (1930), Twitty and Schwind (1931), Dempster (1933), and Moore (1939). At metamorphosis the animals have attained a length of 48–55 mm.

2. *Ambystoma tigrinum.*—No stage series for this form has been worked out. The H-stages for *A. maculatum* can be applied roughly to this form if one uses gill and tail development for identification but disregards limb development. The forelimb buds that appear in *A. maculatum* in stages H36–H37 appear in *A. tigrinum* very belatedly, namely, in the feeding stage, which corresponds to H46 for *A. maculatum*. Another profound difference between the two forms is found in their growth rates. Adults of *A. tigrinum* are of approximately double the size of *A. maculatum*, and this difference is reflected in the higher

TABLE 1

TIMETABLE FOR *A. maculatum*

(At Room Temperature, Approx. 20° C.)

	STAGES											
	H2	H3	H4	H5	H7	H9	H11	H13	H14	H17	H19	H23
Time*.....	0	2	4	6	12–14	34–36	2	$2\frac{1}{2}$	3	$3\frac{1}{2}$	$3\frac{3}{4}$–4	$4\frac{1}{2}$–5

	STAGES										
	H29	H34	H36	H38	H39	H40	H42	H43	H44	H45	H46
Time*.....	7	8	9	12	14	15–16	18–19	20	21	23–24	25

* H3–H9 in hours; from H11 on, in days.

growth rate (increment in length per time unit) of *A. tigrinum* from early stages on. Growth curves for *A. tigrinum* are to be found in Harrison (1929), Stone (1930), Twitty and Schwind (1931), and Moore (1939). As a result of the higher growth rate, maximally fed larvae of *A. tigrinum* are about 100–110 mm. long at metamorphosis, as compared to 48–55 mm. for *A. maculatum*. Both forms, if fed maximally, metamorphose at about the same time (approximately 76 days after fertilization, according to Twitty and Schwind, 1931). Under less favorable conditions the time of metamorphosis of *A. tigrinum* is extremely variable; it may be delayed up to 17 months (Harrison, 1929). Stone (1930) gives 130 days as an average.

The rapid rate of development of *A. tigrinum* is also expressed in the greater speed with which a given H-stage is reached, as compared to *A. maculatum*. According to Moore (1939) and my own limited data, the rates of development compare approximately as shown in Table 2.

21

Hatching takes place in approximately the same stage as in *A. maculatum*, which is the equivalent of H40–H42 (13–14 days). However, the forelimbs, at that stage, are barely visible buds; they are comparable to those of H37 for *A. maculatum*.

3. *Ambystoma opacum.*—No stage series has been worked out. Growth proceeds more slowly than in *A. maculatum*. Growth curves in Twitty and Elliott (1934, p. 284) and Moore (1939).

4. *Other urodeles.*—A stage series for the common American red-spotted newt, *Diemictylus viridescens*, has been prepared by Fankhauser (unpublished). The common European newt, *Triturus taeniatus* (=vulgaris) has been staged by several workers. The old "Normentafel" by Glaesner (1925) is still in use, though it is not very satisfactory because the stages are too far apart and the drawings often make a diagnosis difficult. More recently, a series has been worked out that conforms to the *Ambystoma* series of Harrison. The early period, up to stage 36 has been staged by Rotmann (1940). Good drawings of

TABLE 2

DAYS REQUIRED TO REACH A GIVEN H-STAGE
(At Approx. 20° C.)

	STAGES					
	H11	H23	H32	H39	H41	H46
A. tigrinum..........	1½	3	5–6	8–9	11–12	15–16
A. maculatum........	2	4	7–8	14	16–18	25

the most frequently used tail-bud stages may be found in Sato (1933). The later period, from larval stage 36 to metamorphosis, is covered by the series of Glücksohn (1931). These stages are identified largely on the basis of the development of the limbs and characteristic changes in the relative lengths of the toes. This publication includes a parallel series for the crested newt (*Triturus cristatus*) whose unpigmented eggs have been used frequently for heteroplastic transplantation. A stage series for another widely used European newt, *Triturus alpestris*, was worked out by Knight (1938) and one for *Triturus helveticus* by Gallien and Bidaud (1959). *Pleurodeles waltlii* has been staged by Gallien and Durocher (1957), and the *Axolotl* by Stauffer (1945).

A stage series for the Japanese newt, *Triturus pyrrhogaster*, which is being used also by American and European workers, was published by Okada and Ichikawa (1947, in Japanese). A series up to larval stages (not conforming to the Harrison series) was prepared by Anderson (1943). Twitty and Bodenstein have prepared a stage series for the California newt, *Taricha torosa*, which is published in Rugh (1948).

Rate of development.—Gallien and Durocher (1957) give a comparative timetable for the development of the most widely used urodeles, at 18° C.

(taken, in part, from the authors quoted above). Stauffer (1945) gives corresponding data for the Axolotl.

ORDER Urodela

5. Rana pipiens.—A stage seriation has been published by Shumway (1940) (see Fig. 43). It covers the phase from fertilization to the young tadpole, in which the gills are just overgrown by the operculum and the animal has not fed yet. Twenty-five stages are distinguished. They are conveniently tabulated, together with average body length and age (at 18° C.). This seriation is already widely adopted and will be referred to in the text as Sh1–Sh25.

Rate of development.—The studies of Atlas (1935) and of Moore (1939, 1949b) give full information on this point (see also Shumway, 1940).[3] In Moore's paper the rate of development (in hours) in terms of Sh-stages is given for four different temperatures (15.3°, 18.6°, 19.8°, 26° C.). The following table includes Moore's figures for "room temperature," 19.8° C.

TABLE 3

RATES OF DEVELOPMENT FOR FOUR SPECIES OF Rana
(Time in Hours after First Cleavage; at 19.8° C.; from Moore, 1939, 1942b)

Stage	R. pipiens	R. palustris	R. sylvatica	R. catesbeiana
Sh3	0	0	0	0
Sh10	20–24	20–24	16–20	23
Sh11	25	29.5	20–23	....
Sh12	29–37.5	35	23–26	35
Sh13	38–44	38–43	37.7	42
Sh14	43.5–48	46–55	37.7	48–60
Sh15	50–54.5	55	40.5	60
Sh16	51–58	61–64	40–45	....
Sh17	60–69	66–74	....	83
Sh18	70–84	80–83	50	87–114
Sh18	85–96	95–98	66	120
Sh20	95–103	105–106	72–87	131

OTHER DATA ON NORMAL DEVELOPMENT

First movements: Sh18.

First heartbeat: Sh19.

Hatching: Sh18 (Moore, 1940b); Sh20 (Shumway, 1940).

Spontaneous swimming: Sh21.

Feeding: Sh25.

Metamorphosis in the field: July, i.e., 13–16 weeks after egg-laying (Wright, 1914).

Temperature tolerance: See Table 4.

6. Rana sylvatica.—In the stage series for this form by Pollister and Moore (1937) the period from tne uncleaved egg to the beginning of the overgrowth

[3] Moore (1949b) has shown that intraspecific differences in rates of development exist between northern and southern populations.

of the operculum is divided into 23 stages, comparable to Sh1–Sh23 for *R. pipiens*. They will be designated as PM1—PM23. (See Figure 44.)

Rate of development.—Development rate is considerably faster than that of *R. pipiens*. See Table 3.

OTHER DATA ON NORMAL DEVELOPMENT

First motility: PM18.

First heartbeat: PM19.

Hatching: PM20-PM21.

Spontaneous swimming: PM23.

Metamorphosis in the field: Early in July, that is, 14–16 weeks after egg-laying (Wright, 1914).

Temperature tolerance: See Table 4.

7. *Rana palustris.*—No stage series is available.

Rate of development.—At 19.8° C.; see Table 3. For rates for other tem-

TABLE 4

TEMPERATURE TOLERANCE FOR AMPHIBIANS (IN CENTRIGRADE)

(From Moore, 1940*b*, 1949*a*)

	R. pipiens	*R. sylvatica*	*R. palustris*	*R. catesbeiana*	*Ambystoma maculatum*
Low........	5°	2.5°	7°	15°	3.5°
High........	28°	24°	30°	32°	23°

peratures see Moore (1939). The development is somewhat slower than that of *R. pipiens*.

Hatching: Stage PM17–PM18.

Metamorphosis in the field: In August, that is, 14–17 weeks after egg-laying (Wright, 1914).

Temperature tolerance: See Table 4.

8. *Rana catesbeiana.*—No stage series is available. The eggs are laid late in the season, and metamorphosis takes place two years later.

Rate of development.—See Table 3. For rates for other temperatures see Moore 1942*b*.

Hatching: Stages PM17–PM18.

Temperature tolerance: See Table 4.

9. *Other Anura.*—An elaborate normal table for *Xenopus laevis* has been prepared by Nieuwkoop and Faber (1956). It includes a table comparing this stage series with that of other anurans, age data at 22°–24°, data on rearing *Xenopus,* and an extensive bibliography of stage series for amphibians in general.

24

BIBLIOGRAPHY

ANDERSON, P. L. 1943. The normal development of *Triturus pyrrhogaster*. Anat. Rec., **86:**58.

ATLAS, M. 1935. The effect of temperature on the development of *Rana pipiens*. Physiol. Zoöl., **8:**290.

DEMPSTER, W. T. 1933. Growth in *Amblystoma punctatum* during the embryonic and early larval period. Jour. Exper. Zool., **64:**495.

DuSHANE, G. P., and HUTCHINSON, C. 1941. The effect of temperature on the development of form and behavior in amphibian embryos. Jour. Exper. Zool., **87:**245.

GALLIEN, L., and BIDAUD, O. 1959. Table chronologique du développement chez *Triturus helveticus* Razoumowsky. Bull. Soc. Zool. France, **84:**22.

———— and DUROCHER, M. 1957. Table chronologique du développement chez *Pleurodeles waltlii* Michah. Bull. Biol., **91:**97.

GLÄSNER, L. 1925. Normentafel zur Entwicklung des gemeinen Wassermolches Molge vulgaris. Keibel's Normentafeln, No. 14.

GLÜCKSOHN, S. 1931. Äussere Entwicklung der Extremitäten und Stadieneinteilung der Larvenperiode von *Triton taeniatus* Leyd. und *Triton cristatus* Laur. Arch. f. Entw'mech., **125:**341.

HARRISON, R. G. 1929. Correlations in the development and growth of the eye studied by means of heteroplastic transplantation. Arch. f. Entw'mech., **120:**1.

KNIGHT, F. C. E. 1938. Die Entwicklung von *Triton alpestris* bei verschiedenen Temperaturen, mit Normentafel. Arch. f. Entw'mech., **137:**461.

MOORE, J. A. 1939. Temperature tolerance and rates of development in the eggs of Amphibia. Ecology, **20:**459.

————. 1940*a*. Adaptive differences in the egg membranes of frogs. Amer. Nat., **74:**89.

————. 1940*b*. Stenothermy and eurythermy of animals in relation to habitat. *Ibid.*, p. 188.

————. 1942*a*. The role of temperature in speciation of frogs. Biol. Symposia, **6:**189.

————. 1942*b*. Embryonic temperature tolerance and rate of development in *Rana catesbeiana*. Biol. Bull., **83:**375.

————. 1949*a*. Patterns of evolution in the genus *Rana*. In G. JEPSEN, G. SIMPSON, E. MAYR (eds.), Genetics, paleontology and evolution, pp. 315–78. Princeton, N.J.: Princeton University Press.

————. 1949*b*. Geographic variation of adaptive characters in *Rana pipiens* Schreber. Evolution, **3:**1.

NIEUWKOOP, P. D., and FABER, J. 1956. Normal table of *Xenopus laevis* Daudin. Amsterdam: North-Holland Pub. Co.

OKADA, Y. K., and ICHIKAWA, M. 1947. A new normal table for the development of *Triturus pyrrhogaster* Boie. Exper. Morphol. (Tokyo), **3:**1. (In Japanese.)

POLLISTER, A. W., and MOORE, J. A. 1937. Tables for the normal development of *Rana sylvatica*. Anat. Rec., **68:**489.

ROTMANN, E. 1940. Die Bedeutung der Zellgrösse für die Entwicklung der Amphibienlinse. Arch. f. Entw'mech., **140:**124.

RUGH, R. 1948. Experimental embryology: A Manual of Techniques and Procedures. Minneapolis: Burgess Pub. Co.

SATO, T. 1933. Über die Determination des fetalen Augenspaltes bei *Triton taeniatus*. Arch. f. Entw'mech., **128:**342.

SHUMWAY, W. 1940. Stages in the normal development of *Rana pipiens*. I. External form. Anat. Rec., **78:**139.

STAUFFER, E. 1945. Versuche zur experimentellen Herstellung haploider Axolotl-Merogone. Rev. Suisse de Zool., **52:**232.

STONE, L. S. 1930. Heteroplastic transplantation of eyes between the larvae of two species of Amblystoma. Jour. Exper. Zool., **55:**193.

TWITTY, V. C., and ELLIOTT, H. A. 1934. The relative growth of the amphibian eye, studied by means of transplantation. Jour. Exper. Zool., **68:**247.

—— and SCHWIND, J. L. 1931. The growth of eyes and limbs transplanted heteroplastically between two species of Amblystoma. Jour. Exper. Zool., **59**:61.

WRIGHT, A. H. 1914. Life-histories of the *Anura* of Ithaca, New York. Pub. Carnegie Inst. Washington, No. 197.

c) REARING AND FEEDING OF LARVAE

Rearing.—Mass cultures may be kept in large finger bowls, crystallizing dishes, or large paraffined paper cups of adequate size. Overcrowding should be carefully avoided. Water plants (*Elodea, Vallisneria*) help to keep the cultures in good condition. Water should be changed only when it gets turbid. Tap water should be boiled and allowed to stand for several hours before larvae are placed in it. In some localities tap water contains toxic agents; in this case, spring or pond water must be used.

Urodele larvae will snap at any moving object. They are likely to mutilate each other by biting off gills or limbs, particulary when they are crowded and not fed optimally. Therefore, all valuable specimens, such as operated animals and larvae which are destined for use in regeneration experiments, should be reared singly from early feeding stages on. Paraffined paper cups of adequate size are the most economical containers.

Precautions at metamorphosis.—Metamorphosis is a critical stage for both anuran and urodele larvae. The animals do not feed during this period and become weak unless they have been fed well before the onset of metamorphosis. Facilities for crawling on land must be provided early enough to prevent them from drowning. It is best to prepare special tanks for metamorphosis and to transfer into these all old larvae which show signs of metamorphosis (color changes, large hind limbs in *Urodela;* emergence of one forelimb and tail resorption in *Anura*). In these tanks the water should be only 1–2 inches deep, and an incline which rises above the water level should be built either of pebbles or by tilting a glass plate or a glass dish.

Feeding of urodele larvae.—Urodele larvae begin to feed in stages corresponding to H46, when all yolk reserves are used up. They are carnivorous, and the young larvae feed only on live material, which moves in front of their eyes and thus attracts their attention. Older larvae rely more on their sense of smell and will take small bits of meat. Small ostracods, daphnia, and other crustaceans are an excellent food for very small larvae. *Enchytrae* ("white worms," *Enchytraeus albidus,* an oligochaete) are equally suitable and available at all times. They may be obtained from aquarium dealers or pet shops. They are best kept in moist humus in a dark, cool room (not warmer than 20° C.) and can be cultured easily in the following way: Fill a large earthen pot or culture dish with moist humus, about 3 inches deep. Add a worm culture of at least 2 quarts. Cover it with a lid. Feed the worms with white bread, cereals, or boiled potatoes, soaked in milk. Scatter the food about or place it where the worms are congregated and cover it with about an inch of humus. Remove all food particles that begin to decay; replace them by fresh food. In such cultures, worms of all sizes will be found (further details in Blount, 1937).

Special attention should be paid to the feeding of very young larvae when they first begin to feed. Some larvae are slow and reluctant to take their first food. In such cases it is necessary to prod and "condition" them patiently; if they go without food for several days, they are likely to swallow air bubbles at the water surface, which usually ends fatally. The following procedure is recommended: Select the very smallest *Enchytrae* worms; this is done by spreading humus crumbs and food particles from a culture of *Enchytrae* in a Petri dish under water. The worms begin to wriggle vigorously, and the smallest ones can be picked up with a watchmaker forceps, under the binocular microscope or with the aid of a Beebe loupe. Move the worm slowly in front of the eyes of the larva to elicit the snapping reaction, or drop the worm in front of the larva. If the larva turns away, repeat your offering. Feed several worms in this way.

Urodele larvae are voracious eaters and should be fed abundantly by placing a number of worms of adequate size in the dish. As the larvae grow, larger worms and greater quantities should be fed, about every other day. Remove dead worms (*Enchytrae* die within a few hours when submerged in water). Larvae raised exclusively on *Enchytrae* may develop abnormal hind legs. Therefore it is advisable to feed older larvae with small bits of raw liver or beef or pieces of earthworm.

Feeding of anuran tadpoles.—The feeding habits of anuran tadpoles are entirely different from those of urodeles. The tadpoles are equipped with horny teeth and are omnivorous; they rasp off algae from the walls of the aquarium or from water plants; they feed on dead organisms, etc. Many different food materials have been recommended for laboratory feeding: Pablum; pellets of rabbit food; canned boiled spinach (wash several times); leafy Romaine lettuce, boiled for 3 hours (decant water); boiled meat (finely minced liver, beef, or frog muscle); or a combination of these. The tadpoles feed almost continuously, and their growth and metamorphosis can be speeded up considerably by optimal feeding. Excess food in the container, however, leads to turbidity in the water; therefore it is advisable to feed rather frequently and not to give too much food at a time. Remove all debris carefully. We have had very satisfactory results with the feeding of canned boiled spinach. It can be stored easily in a refrigerator and requires no preparation except washing before use. It is one of the cleanest food materials. If only a few leaves are fed at a time, the water does not get turbid. The formation of kidney stones as a result of an exclusive diet of spinach (Briggs and Davidson, 1942) does not occur until late in development, that is, after the termination of the thyroxin and lithium experiments outlined in this *Manual*.

Operated embryos suffer occasionally from edema, particularly in tail-bud stages. Edematous blebs appear on the flank or on the ventral side. Such animals usually die after several days and should be fixed in early stages of edema if they are valuable material. Sometimes puncturing of the vesicle with a fine glass needle saves the animal (narcotize the animal if necessary).

Fungus infections (*Saprolegnia*) are not infrequent in urodele cultures and are difficult to get rid of. They appear as fine sticky threads, first on gills and legs and eventually all over the body, and are usually fatal. Detwiler and McKennon (1929) recommend a bath of Mercurochrome (di-brom-oxy-mercuri-fluorescin). Animals are kept for several days in a concentration of 1:500,000–1:1,000,000. The molds usually slough off after 2–3 days. Effective concentrations and lengths of exposure should be tried out for each instance. Pet shops sell other good disinfectants.

Young urodele larvae that are not properly fed or are slow in catching food sometimes swallow air bubbles. Occasionally they fill their stomachs with air and float on the surface. This condition is, of course, critical, and the larvae will die of starvation unless the air is removed. Animals placed in shallow water with plenty of food usually get rid of the air bubbles. They can also be removed either by puncturing the stomach with a glass needle or a fine steel knife or by squeezing out the air through the mouth, holding the animal cautiously with one pair of watchmaker forceps and pinching behind the air bubble with another forceps.

BIBLIOGRAPHY

BLOUNT, R. T. 1937. Cultivation of *Enchytraeus albidus*. In P. S. GALTSOFF (ed.), Culture methods for invertebrate animals. Ithaca, N.Y.: Comstock Pub. Co.

BRIGGS, R., and DAVIDSON, M. 1942. Some effects of spinach-feeding on *Rana pipiens* tadpoles. Jour. Exper. Zool., **90**:401.

DETWILER, S. R., and McKENNON, G. E. 1929. Mercurochrome (di-brom-oxy-mercuri-fluorescin) as a fungicidal agent in the growth of amphibian embryos. Anat. Rec., **41**:205.

2. EXPERIMENTAL OVULATION BY HYPOPHYSIS INJECTION AND ARTIFICIAL INSEMINATION

a) Anura

It is now possible to obtain eggs at almost any time of the year, as a result of our increased knowledge of the control of reproduction by the anterior lobe of the hypophysis. R. Rugh (1934–48) has worked out the standard technique on which the following directions are largely based.

In *Anura,* insemination is external. Male and female go into amplexus. The eggs are inseminated externally, immediately after they have passed through the cloaca. The routine procedure for obtaining fertile eggs is to induce ovulation, strip the eggs into a sperm suspension, and submerge them in water 5–10 minutes later to allow the membranes to swell.

The following points are of importance for obtaining optimal results:

1. *Source of anterior lobe substance.*—So far, fresh frog pituitary gland is the only reliable and adequately standardized source for the gonadotropic principle effective in frogs. Implants and extracts of mammalian anterior lobe were unsuccessful (Creaser and Gorbman, 1939).

2. *Size of frogs (Rana pipiens).*—Both donors and recipients must be fully mature. Do not use females under 75 mm. or males under 70 mm. in body length.

3. *Condition of frogs.*—It is important to use only specimens (for donors and recipients) that are in excellent condition. The pituitaries of frogs that are held in room temperature for a long time, starved, or otherwise kept under inadequate conditions lose their potency.

4. *Temperature.*—It is advisable to keep the frogs in a cold room ($4°$–$15°$)

TABLE 5

EFFECTIVE DOSES FOR OVULATION (*R. pipiens*)

	September–December	January–February	March–April
No. of ♀ pituitaries required..........	5–6	3–5	2–3

before treatment. Particularly, recipient females must not be kept at room temperature.

5. *Dosage.*—The dosage has been standardized for *R. pipiens* implants into *R. pipiens* (Rugh, 1948; see Table 5). The number of pituitaries to be injected varies with the season. Rugh found that the pituitaries of mature females are twice as potent as those of mature males. If ♂ glands are used, the doses have to be doubled. Injections during the months immediately following the natural breeding season (April, May) are usually less successful.

The size and physiological potency of different hypophyses, as well as the responsiveness of individual recipients, vary considerably, so that the foregoing figures give only approximate values. It is therefore advisable to inject two or more females for each experiment or demonstration. The effect of injections is cumulative, and it is usually possible to bring a "refractory" female to ovulation by administering a second injection 2 days after a first unsuccessful injection.

Material

hypodermic syringe, 2 cc.

hypodermic needle, No. 18 or 20

29

dissecting instruments, including strong and fine scissors and watchmaker
forceps
section dishes and watch glasses
finger bowls or Petri dishes
battery jars or aquariums with lids or wire coverings to keep the recipients
1/10 Holtfreter solution or spring or pond water for dilution of sperm fluid
a Beebe binocular magnifying glass is helpful in the dissection of the hypophysis

Procedure (for R. pipiens)[4]

1. Prepare as many battery or glass jars as there are females to be injected.
Cover the bottom with water, about 1 inch deep. Cover the jars with heavy
glass lids or wire covering.

2. Select two or more females as recipients. Hold them ready in a small cage.

3. *Dissection of the pituitary glands from the donors* (Fig. 2).—Insert one
blade of a strong pair of scissors into the mouth at the angle of the jaws and
decapitate the frogs by a transverse cut behind the tympanic membrane. Be
sure not to cut more anteriorly. Pith the spinal cord and discard the body.
Wash the head and remove all blood. Turn the head upside down. Dissect and
clean away the skin of the oral cavity and thus expose the base of the skull.
Locate the ⊥-shaped parasphenoid bone. Make two cuts through the floor of

[4] For data on other *Anura* see Rugh (1948).

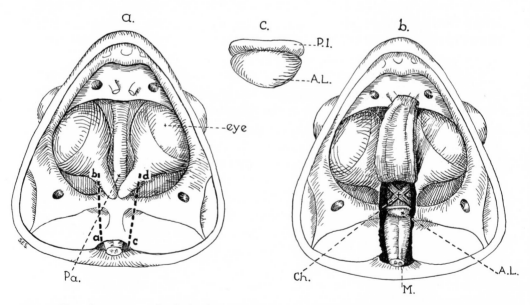

Fig. 2.—Hypophysectomy. *a*, head of a frog, ventral view. *Pa* = parasphenoid bone. *b*, ventral view; brain
and hypophysis exposed. *A.L.* = anterior lobe; *Ch* = optic chiasma; *M* = medull oblongata. *c*, hypophysis
isolated. *A.L.* = anterior lobe; *P.I.* = pars intermedia.

the skull, from the cranial cavity toward the eyes (*ab* and *cd* in Fig. 2, *a*), by inserting the pointed blade of a fine pair of scissors into the foramen magnum or the spinal canal. Do not injure the brain tissue. With a pair of forceps carefully deflect the triangular piece of bone, thus exposing the ventral aspect of the brain (Fig. 2, *b*). Locate the hindbrain, the infundibulum, and the optic chiasma. The anterior lobe of the hypophysis can now be recognized by its pinkish color. Either it is in its normal position (attached to the infundibulum, posterior to the optic chiasma), or it adheres to the deflected bone. Grasp the gland with a pair of fine forceps and place it in $\frac{1}{10}$ Holtfreter solution in a watch glass. (Make your first dissections under the binocular microscope or with a loupe.) The anterior lobe is pinkish and bean-shaped. Attached to its anterior straight edge is usually a slender whitish body, the *pars intermedia* and *pars nervosa* (Fig. 2, *c*). Remove this tissue with two pairs of watchmaker forceps. Dissect as many glands as are required according to Table 5 (p. 29); collect them all in the watch glass.

4. *Injection.*—Draw the glands into the barrel of the syringe before you insert the injection needle. Hold the female that is to be injected in your left hand and insert the needle through the flank skin into the body cavity. Push the needle forward and downward under the skin, and not medially, to avoid injury to the viscera. Inject and then withdraw the needle cautiously; while you withdraw, pinch the skin at the needle entrance to avoid outflow of hypophysis material. To insure that no gland material is lost by adhering to the needle, squirt water through the syringe and inject all material that is recovered in this way.

5. Place the female in a jar. Label the jar and indicate date and dose. Preferably keep it in a cool place, not higher than 20° C.

6. *Test of ovulation by "stripping."*—At room temperature most of the eggs should have ovulated in 24–48 hours after the injection, if the above doses are applied. Test ovulation in the following way: Bend the legs forward and hold the frog in your right hand. Press gently in the direction of the cloaca. In this way eggs will be forced out without injury to the frog. If a string of eggs appears, release the pressure at once, place the female back in the container, and prepare the sperm fluid. If only liquid or jelly oozes out, then ovulation has not yet taken place, and another test should be made 12–24 hours later. If no eggs are obtained, a second injection should be made.

7. *Preparation of the sperm fluid.*—The males of *R. pipiens* usually contain functional sperm throughout the year, so that it is not necessary to give them hypophysis injections. Prepare a dish with 20 cc. of 10 per cent Holtfreter solution or 0.1 per cent amphibian Ringer solution or pond or spring water. Do not use tap water or distilled water. A quantity of 10 cc. per pair of testes is usually recommended for sperm suspensions, but even a tenfold dilution of this suspension still gives optimal results.

Decapitate and pith 2 large males, not under 70 mm. in length. Dissect out both pairs of testes (yellow, oval bodies, located near the anterior borders of the kidneys). Clean them of adhering blood and tissue and macerate them thoroughly with forceps and scissors until a milky suspension is obtained. Allow it to stand for 5–10 minutes, during which time the spermatozoa become active. Check under the microscope whether active, motile sperms are present.

8. *Stripping and insemination.*—Divide the sperm suspension among 2–3 finger bowls or large Petri dishes so that the bottom of the dish is just covered. Hold the female as in section 6 and strip the eggs directly into the sperm fluid by slow, continued pressure. The eggs will ooze out in a string. Line them up in rows or in a spiral so that all eggs are exposed to the sperm and are not clustered. Shake the dish gently to insure complete fertilization. After 5–10 minutes flood the dish with the same medium that was used for sperm suspension, rinse and wash the eggs, and let them stand submerged in clean water. The jelly membranes will swell slowly. A successful insemination is usually indicated after about 1 hour by the rotation of the eggs, as a result of which all dark animal poles move upward. The first cleavage is to be expected $2\frac{1}{2}$ hours after insemination, at room temperature. If eggs are clustered, they should be separated with a scalpel. Do not keep more than 30–40 eggs in a finger bowl.

9. *"Fractionated" stripping.*—Eggs remain viable in the oviduct for some time (see below) if the females are kept at a low temperature (10°–15° C.). It is therefore possible to obtain eggs from the same female over a period of several days. Stripping is simply interrupted when the desired number of eggs is recovered, and the female is returned to the cold room.

VIABILITY OF EGGS, SPERM, AND PITUITARY GLANDS (*R. pipiens*)

Eggs.—Eggs will remain fully viable and fertilizable and will give an optimal percentage of normal development for 3–4 days after the onset of ovulation if the females are kept at 10°–15° C. From then on, the percentage of fertilization and of normal development decreases steadily (Zimmerman and Rugh, 1941).

Sperm.—According to Moore and Barth (personal communication), a sperm suspension of 10 pairs of testes in 150 cc. of 0.1 per cent amphibian Ringer at 15° C. retained its fertilizability for 20 hours. However, it is always advisable to use fresh suspensions.

Pituitary glands.—According to Rugh (1937), dissected glands retain their potency for a long period if kept in absolute alcohol in the refrigerator. Dilute the alcohol to 35 per cent before injection.

b) Urodela

In the urodeles, the male deposits a spermatophore after a prolonged court-ship; the female takes it up into a gland of the cloaca (spermotheca), where the spermatozoa remain functional for a long period. The eggs are insem-inated individually while they pass through the cloaca. The general practice for obtaining fertile eggs outside the breeding season is to inject only the fe-males and to rely for fertilization on the presence of functional spermatozoa in the spermotheca. The eggs laid by *Diemictylus viridescens, Triturus pyrrho-gaster* and *Taricha torosa* females, following hyophysis injection are fertilized in most instances, but occasionally one encounters a female that lays unfer-tilized eggs. Hypophyses of *Diemictylus viridescens* as well as of *R. pipiens* can be used; the latter are preferable because they are larger and easier to dissect. *Diemictylus* females respond also to mammalian pituitary extracts: phyone (a growth-stimulating fraction) and hebin (a gonadotropic fraction; Adams, 1934). However, the dosage has not been standardized. We recom-mend the use of fresh *R. pipiens* glands for *D. viridescens* (Kaylor, 1937; Griffiths, 1941; Fankhauser, personal communication).[5] The females are kept in the refrigerator at about 10° C. between the day of collection and the first implantation. This keeps the ovaries in good condition for at least 2 months. At room temperature ovaries deteriorate in about 2 weeks. The procedure of injection is the same as in frogs, with slight modifications. Whereas in the frog a large number of eggs are ovulated almost simultaneously, the eggs of the newts are laid singly over a period of several weeks. Therefore, in order to obtain a continuous egg production, it is advisable to inject several doses with an interval of 1–2 days between the injections. The standard procedure in Dr. Fankhauser's laboratory is to inject a single *R. pipiens* hypophysis on the first day and another single hypophysis on the third day. Two hypophyses were found sufficient to stimulate ovulation at any time between October and May. The first eggs are usually laid on the third to sixth day following the first implantation, and the egg-laying period lasts between 6 and 14 days on the average. It is advisable to inject a considerable number of females for each experiment, since the number of females that do not respond to the injections or that lay unfertilized eggs is rather high (30–40 per cent). The hypophyses are usually implanted under the skin of the lower jaws. Injected females should be placed in jars or tanks in which they can swim around comfortably and should be amply provided with fresh *Elodea* or *Vallisneria*. The eggs are de-posited on the leaves of these water plants (see p. 17). For collection of eggs, take out all water plants each day and inspect each leaf. Remove the eggs carefully with a watchmaker forceps.

Triturus pyrrhogaster may be treated in the same way (Streett, 1940). In

---

[5] I am indebted to Dr. Gerhard Fankhauser for making available to me his records of injections and for the communication of certain technical details.

class experiments we obtained from 15 to 150 eggs per female after 2 injections of 2 *R. pipiens* glands each, on 2 successive days or with a 1-day interval between the 2 injections.

Certain experiments, for instance, hybridization, require artificial insemination. The eggs cannot be stripped but must be recovered from the oviduct. Prepare a number of Petri dishes laid out with moist filter paper ("moist chambers") and clean microscope slides. Decapitate and pith several males and females. Dissect the testes and the (usually pigmented) vasa efferentia and macerate them thoroughly in 10 cc. of pond or spring water or $\frac{1}{10}$ Holtfreter solution. Dissect out the oviducts, place them on glass plates, and very carefully slit them or cut them open and set the eggs free. They are soft and delicate and must be handled with utmost caution. Mount them singly on the slides; do not moisten them. With a fine pipette, drop a few drops of the sperm suspension over each egg so that it is well coated. Place the slides in the moist chambers for 5–10 minutes, then submerge them in water. After the membranes are swollen, rinse off the sperm suspension and remove the eggs from the slides with a scalpel. If artificial hybridization is planned, discard all eggs found in the cloaca, because they may be fertilized.

BIBLIOGRAPHY (*a–b*)

ADAMS, A. E. 1934. The gonad- and thyroid-stimulating potencies of phyone and hebin. Anat. Rec., **59**:349.

CREASER, C. W., and GORBMAN, A. 1939. Species specificity of the gonadotropic factors in vertebrates. Quart. Rev. Biol., **14**:311.

GRIFFITHS, R. B. 1941. Triploidy (and haploidy) in the newt, *Triturus viridescens,* induced by refrigeration of fertilized eggs. Genetics, **26**:69.

KAYLOR, C. T. 1937. Experiments on androgenesis in the newt, *Triturus viridescens.* Jour. Exper. Zool., **76**:375.

RUGH, R. 1934. Induced ovulation and artificial fertilization in the frog. Biol. Bull., **66**:22.

———. 1937. Ovulation induced out of season. Science, **85**:588.

———. 1948. Experimental embryology: A manual of techniques and procedures. Minneapolis: Burgess Pub. Co.

STREETT, J. C. 1940. Experiments on the organization of the unsegmented egg of *Triturus pyrrhogaster.* Jour. Exper. Zool., **85**:383.

ZIMMERMAN, L., and RUGH, R. 1941. Effect of age on the development of the egg of the leopard frog, *Rana pipiens.* Jour. Morphol., **68**:329.

3. PREPARATION FOR EXPERIMENTS

a) CULTURE MEDIA

Special culture media have been devised for use during the operations and for rearing of early embryos and of isolated embryonic parts.

1. The standard culture medium is the "Holtfreter solution" or "Standard solution" (Holtfreter, 1931). It is a modified dilute Ringer solution which was originally designed for the culturing of isolated fragments of gastrulae and other early embryos. Its composition is shown in Table 6.

The introduction of this medium signaled an important advance in methodology. Isolates, reared in this solution over prolonged periods, will undergo cellular differentiation and morphogenesis (utilizing their yolk content for nutrition); hence new possibilities were opened up for the study of problems of differentiation and induction.

In all media, osmotic pressure and the pH are of prime importance. The Holtfreter solution is isotonic, but its pH (above 8) is somewhat higher than optimal. Therefore, Holtfreter now reduces the $NaHCO_3$ buffer to 0.02, which gives a stable pH at 7.5 (personal communication). If the Tris-HCl buffer is used (see below under 3), it is advisable not to dispense with $NaHCO_3$ entirely.

TABLE 6

COMPOSITION OF HOLTFRETER AND
AMPHIBIAN RINGER SOLUTION

(In Gm/Liter)

Solution	NaCl	KCl	CaCl₂	NaHCO₃
Holtfreter..........	3.5	0.05	0.1	0.02
Amphibian Ringer..	6.5	0.14	0.12	0.1

Add bicarbonate after the solution has cooled down or make up 2 solutions separately.

The full-strength Holtfreter solution facilitates wound-healing. It is now a generally adopted practice to *perform all operations in this solution* and to leave the embryos in it until the wound is completely healed or until the transplant is healed in. However, prolonged culturing of early embryos in this medium is detrimental; for instance, early amphibian gastrulae will exogastrulate if kept in full-strength Holtfreter solution after removal of the vitelline membrane, and neurulation is impeded. Hence, early embryos have to be transferred to a *10 per cent Holtfreter solution* after wound-healing is completed. However, isolated parts must be reared in the full-strength solution. Neurulae and older embryos tolerate full-strength solution.

Use distilled water for preparing sterile solution. Prepare the solution without $NaHCO_3$ and autoclave. $NaHCO_3$ has to be sterilized separately by dry heat, and then added, to prevent its precipitation. Allow the solution to cool off before using it. For use of a class of 8–12 students it is best to prepare the concentrated stock solution in 2- or 3-liter flasks. It is not advisable to prepare too large quantities, because the solutions deteriorate. Add antibiotics before use (see below).

2. *The Niu-Twitty Solution.*—This solution (Niu and Twitty, 1953) is pre-

35

pared in three parts, as shown in the accompanying tabulation. The three solutions are boiled separately and mixed after cooling. The pH is approximately 7.6. The medium can be used for rearing of embryos and of isolates.

SOLUTION A (500 cc. dist. water)		SOLUTION B (250 cc. dist. water)		SOLUTION C (250 cc. dist. water)	
NaCl.	3,400 mg.	Na$_2$HPO$_4$.	110 mg.	NaHCO$_3$.	200 mg.
KCl.	50	KH$_2$PO$_4$.	20		
Ca(NO$_3$)·4H$_2$O. .	80				
MgSO$_4$.	100				

3. *Steinberg medium.*—The salt combination (M. Steinberg, 1957) is taken over from Niu-Twitty (see under 2), but the buffers are replaced by a Tris-HCl buffer (Tris available through Sigma Chemical Co., St. Louis) which adjusts to a pH of 7.4 (see accompanying formula). The entire solution

FORMULA

17 per cent NaCl.	20 ml.	1.00 per cent N HCl.	4 ml.
0.5 per cent KCl.	10 ml.	Tris.	560 mg.
0.8 per cent Ca(NO$_3$)·4H$_2$O. . . .	10 ml.	Glass distilled H$_2$O.	946 ml.
2.05 per cent MgSO$_4$·7H$_2$O. . . .	10 ml.		

s made up in one flask and autoclaved. It is suggested that the medium be diluted for the rearing of whole embryos. In this instance, it is essential *not to dilute the buffer.*

Antibiotics.—It is recommended that streptomycin and penicillin be added to the culture media in the following concentrations: Add 1.2 cc. of a 0.02 per cent solution of *streptomycin sulfate* to each liter of concentrated or dilute culture medium (must be made up fresh before use). Dilute 1,000 units of penicillin in 1 cc. of distilled water. Add 1 cc. of this solution to each liter of culture medium.

BIBLIOGRAPHY

HOLTFRETER, J. 1931. Über die Aufzucht isolierter Teile des Amphibienkeimes. Arch. f. Entw'mech., **124**:404.
NIU, M. C., and TWITTY, V. C. 1953. The differentiation of gastrula ectoderm in medium conditioned by axial mesoderm. Proc. Nat. Acad. Sci., **39**:985.
STEINBERG, M. 1957. In: Carnegie Institution of Washington Year Book 56, p. 347.

b) STERILIZATION MEASURES

The removal of the jelly membranes and of the vitelline membrane preparatory to the operation deprives the embryo of its major defense against bacterial infection. The operation itself disrupts the surface coat that serves as an additional protection against infection, and the embryo is thus laid wide open to bacterial invasion until the wound is healed. The danger of infection is enhanced further by the use of agar as a bottom layer for operation and culture dishes; agar is very well suited as a substrate for the growing embryos but, unfortunately, also as a substrate for bacteria. For these reasons a thorough sterilization of all instruments, glassware, and culture media is imperative for work on gastrulae, neurula, and tail-bud stages. Older embryos are less susceptible. For sterilization procedures during operations see page 43.

Glassware.—Culture dishes, Erlenmeyer flasks, pipettes, etc., should be sterilized in a hot oven at 180° for an hour. Glass needles are too delicate to be sterilized in this way. It is advisable for each student to have a beaker with boiling water on the operation table and to dip the needle in the water before use. Prepare fresh needles for each operation session.

Metal instruments.—Watchmaker forceps, needles, platinum wire loops, knives, etc., should be cleaned carefully and placed in 70 per cent alcohol in a beaker or glass jar whose bottom is covered with cotton. Pull these instruments quickly through a flame (alcohol burner, if no gas is available) before using them. Be sure that no alcohol drops adhere to the instruments.

Always keep all dishes (except those for instruments) covered. For flasks containing culture fluids use of an inverted beaker as a lid is preferable to a cotton stopper.

For sterilization of culture media and use of antibiotics see page 35.

c) THE REMOVAL OF EGG MEMBRANES (DECAPSULATION)

All amphibian eggs are inclosed in a vitelline membrane and in a number of gelatinous envelopes. Their number and consistency differ in different species. Descriptions, measurements, and illustrations may be found in Wright and Wright (1924), Bishop (1941), and Stebbins (1951). The removal of the membranes is usually done mechanically with forceps. Different forms require different techniques, which are described below. The removal of the vitelline membrane offers particular difficulties in stages prior to neurulation, and in cleavage and morula stages its removal with forceps is practically impossible without serious injury. Steinberg (1957) has described a simple technique of *chemical digestion* of the vitelline membrane that seems to overcome this difficulty. A very small crystal of cysteine hydrochloride is placed close to the surface of the egg and then rapidly flushed away with a stream of fluid from a pipette. The membrane ruptures near the crystal and can then be removed with forceps. It is necessary to gauge the time of exposure and the distance of the crystal from the egg correctly because the embryo itself is easily injured by the treatment. A good deal of practice is necessary before the technique can be applied to valuable material.

Ambystoma.—The eggs of the three species *A. maculatum, A. tigrinum,* and *A. opacum* are approximately equal in size, ranging from $2\frac{1}{2}$ to 3 mm. The vitelline membrane is closely applied to the egg. A second rather tough and

37

perfectly transparent membrane forms a capsule, about 5½–6 mm. in diameter. The space between the vitelline membrane and this capsule is filled with the capsular fluid in which the egg moves freely. The capsule is surrounded by another tough and less transparent membrane, which consists, in *A. maculatum*, of several thin layers. In *A. tigrinum* an additional membrane is found between the two. In all *Ambystoma* species a thin, sticky layer forms the outermost covering. In *A. maculatum* and *A. tigrinum* the eggs are imbedded in a common jelly, which probably originates by coalescence of individual soft jelly layers. The eggs of *A. opacum* are laid singly under leaves, etc. (see p. 16). Their outermost sticky membrane is usually covered with mud particles.

Two pairs of watchmaker forceps with carefully sharpened points are needed for the removal of the membranes. The eggs of *A. maculatum* and *A. tigrinum* are first taken out of their common jell mass; those of *A. opacum*

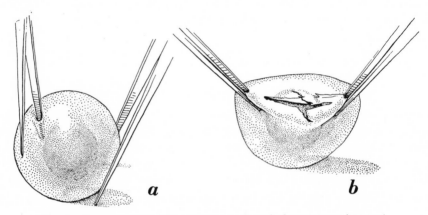

a   *b*

Fig. 3.—Removal of the jelly membranes of an *Ambystoma* egg (see text)

are placed in water and allowed to swell to capacity. The eggs are transferred to a Petri dish or other glass dish. Perform all further manipulations under the low-power binocular dissection microscope. The two outermost layers—the sticky, thin membrane and the outer capsule—can be easily removed together. Next follows the inner capsule, which is under the pressure of the capsular fluid. Remove it in the following way (Fig. 3). Set the forceps, in your right hand, firmly on the glass bottom, with extended prongs, and push the egg against it. Pierce the capsule with one prong of the left forceps (Fig. 3, *a*). Carefully avoid injury to the egg. No fluid can escape because the forceps plug the hole. Next close the left forceps and hold a firm grip on the capsular membrane. Then insert one point of the right forceps into the hole alongside the left forceps (Fig. 3, *b*) and rupture the membrane with a quick jerk of both pairs of forceps in opposite directions. The capsular fluid will then escape, and the egg will pop out, or it can be shaken out.

The *removal of the vitelline membrane* is rather difficult in young stages.

For this purpose the forceps must be sharpened to the finest points possible. The removal is usually unsuccessful in cleavage stages. In blastula and gastrula stages the vitelline membrane is still very closely applied to the egg but can be removed in the following way. Puncture the vitelline membrane over the animal pole with a glass needle or the point of the forceps. A slight injury to the animal pole is inevitable, but small holes usually heal well. The blastocoele fluid escapes, and the embryo will flatten somewhat, or wrinkles will appear on the egg surface. Grasp the vitelline membrane with the left forceps near the hole over the animal pole or over one of the wrinkles, and with the right forceps tear the edge of the membrane next to the left forceps. Tear a large hole by moving both forceps apart. Following removal of all membranes, the egg will collapse. It is very delicate and must be handled with extreme care. If used for operations, it should be washed in several changes of sterile Holtfreter solution and placed in a dish with agar bottom in $\frac{1}{10}$ Holtfreter solution. If the egg was punctured, place it in full Holtfreter solution for a while to facilitate healing. Use sterilized pipettes and dishes and keep all dishes covered. From neurula stages on, the removal of the vitelline membrane offers no difficulties.

Diemictylus.—In the eggs of *Diemictylus viridescens,* the outer capsule, including the outermost sticky membrane, can be removed with little difficulty. However, the pressure of the capsular fluid is considerably greater than in *Ambystoma* eggs, and the removal of the inner capsule is more difficult and requires a different technique. To recover the embryo without injury, it is necessary to tear a large hole in the capsule as soon as the latter is pierced by the forceps. Pull the 2 forceps apart with a rapid, jerky movement. For a short period immediately after fertilization, the tension of the capsular fluid is low, and, if eggs are to be used in cleavage or gastrula stages, they should be decapsulated shortly after they are deposited. Since the successful removal of the inner capsule is difficult and requires some experience, *Diemictylus* embryos in stages preceding the tail-bud stage are not recommended for classroom experiments.

Taricha torosa (Triturus torosus).—Decapsulation of *Taricha* embryos is easy. Cut a hole in the capsule with a pair of fine scissors and remove the embryo with a pipette of appropriate size.

Frogs.—Frog eggs are imbedded in a common jelly mass and individually surrounded by loose jelly layers, which, however, form no tough, elastic capsules. The jelly is not difficult to remove. One may cut it off with forceps or roll the eggs on filter paper. It is difficult to remove the vitelline membrane in early stages up to neurulae without injury to the embryo. Besides, decapsulated anuran eggs are very soft and extremely delicate. Frog gastrulae are therefore not suitable for classroom experiments; but, in embryos from late neurula stages on, all membranes, including the vitelline membrane, can be easily removed with forceps.

39

BIBLIOGRAPHY

BISHOP, S. C. 1941. The salamanders of New York. New York State Mus. Bull. 324. Albany:
University of the State of New York.
STEBBINS, R. C. 1951. Amphibians of western North America. Berkeley: University of Califor-
nia Press.
STEINBERG, M. 1957. In: Carnegie Institution of Washington Year Book 56, p. 348.
WRIGHT, A. H., and WRIGHT, A. A. 1924. A key to the eggs of the *Salientia* east of the
Mississippi River. Amer. Nat., **58**:375.

d) NARCOSIS

Amphibians in tail-bud stages are ciliated and rotate within the capsular
fluid. The ciliary beat is strong enough to keep the animal in slow motion when
it is taken out of the membranes. This may be an impediment in operations.
The only way to hold the embryo tight is to bury it in an agar groove or under
glass bridges.

The first muscular motility begins in stages corresponding to H31 or H32
for *A. maculatum* (see p. 20). From these stages on, the embryos must be narcotized for operations and for recording. Two excellent narcotics are at our
disposal, neither of which has a detrimental effect on the urodele embryo if
applied in proper dosage.

1. *Chloretone* (*acetone chloroform*).—Dissolves rather sparingly in any
culture medium. Shake thoroughly. Keep bottles tightly stoppered and dishes
covered. In most cases a concentration of 1:3,000 will be satisfactory. Old
larvae may require a stronger concentration. It is advisable to try out the effectiveness of the concentration before valuable material is narcotized. Embryos and larvae become immobile within a few minutes and recover within
5–10 minutes. The heart beat should be watched. Its stoppage is a sign of too
high concentration; embryos can be saved if they are transferred immediately
to a normal medium. Embryos may be kept under light narcotization for several days (see p. 139; see also Matthews and Detwiler, 1926).

2. *MS 222.*[6]—This is a methan-sulfonate of meta-amino-benzoic-acid-ethyl-
ester, an isomer of anesthesin (Rothlin, 1932). It is soluble in water and even
less toxic than chloretone. Dissolve it in $\frac{1}{10}$ Holtfreter solution. The animals
recover more rapidly than from chloretone. Copenhaver (1939) finds that the
heart beat is only slightly affected. Concentrations of 1:5,000 or 1:6,000 are
recommended. Again, a normal heart beat is the best indicator for a proper
dosis. Embryos can be kept under light MS anesthesia for several days.

Anuran tadpoles are much more sensitive, and, particularly, older tadpoles
tolerate only low concentrations of MS (1:10,000 or lower) for short periods
(5–10 minutes). It is recommended that anuran tadpoles not be narcotized at
all but that they be placed, for inspection, on a bed of moist cotton under the
binocular microscope.

[6] A product of Sandoz Chemical Works, Inc.

BIBLIOGRAPHY

COPENHAVER, W. M. 1939. Initiation of beat and intrinsic contraction rates in the different parts of the *Amblystoma* heart. Jour. Exper. Zool., **80**:192.

MATTHEWS, S. A., and DETWILER, S. R. 1926. The reactions of *Amblystoma* embryos following prolonged treatment with chloretone. Jour. Exper. Zool., **45**:279.

ROTHLIN, E. 1932. MS 222 (lösliches Anaesthesin), ein Narkotikum für Kaltblüter. Schweiz. med. Wchnschr., **45**:1042.

4. BASIC PROCEDURES FOR OPERATIONS ON AMPHIBIAN EMBRYOS

Operations on Amphibian embryos require manual skill, a steady hand, and patience. However, the final success depends not only on a well-performed operation but to a considerable degree, often underrated by the beginner, on the way in which the delicate embryos are handled before and after the operation; on the use of adequate instruments; and on other technicalities. As is the case in other fields, standard techniques have been worked out for experimental embryology, and they should be adhered to in every detail. This does not imply that the techniques could not be perfected; in fact, improvements are being reported all the time, and the students should be encouraged to try out modifications of their own design. Nevertheless, there are certain basic requirements that cannot be disregarded without risk of failure or of high mortality.

In the following, we list the essential requirements:

1. *Cleanliness.*—General cleanliness and neatness in the laboratory and in the care of living embryos is an absolute necessity.

2. *Handling of eggs before operation.*—The care of the material begins when the egg clusters get into the hands of the experimenter. When collecting eggs in the field, avoid crowding in jars, shaking during transportation, and exposure to heat. *Ambystoma* eggs, which are the most commonly used material for experiments, should be handled in the following way as soon as they arrive in the laboratory: Dip each cluster of eggs briefly in a 1 per cent solution of KOH; use tongs to hold the egg mass. Immediately rinse off the KOH by dipping the cluster in a finger bowl filled with pond or spring or boiled tap water and repeat the washing once or twice. Then take the embryos out of the common jelly, using strong forceps, but leave them in their individual capsules. Next, pipette the eggs into another dish containing a 0.5 per cent solution of *sodium-sulfadiazine* in distilled or boiled tap water and leave them in this solution for 15–30 minutes. (This solution has to be made up fresh each time it is used.) Transfer the eggs to finger bowls or crystallizing dishes with pond or spring or boiled tap water (sulfadiazine precipitate on the jelly capsules does no harm; on the contrary, it may give further protection). Avoid crowding of eggs. Do not cover the dishes. Change water only when it gets turbid.

If there is no time to take the eggs out of the jelly at once, then the large egg masses of *Ambystoma* and frogs should be divided into small batches of 20–30 eggs. If large clusters are left undivided and in insufficient amount of water, the eggs in the center of the mass are liable to die or to develop abnormally.

3. *Temperature.*—Amphibian embryos develop normally only when they are kept within a certain range of temperatures, approximately between 5° and 30° C. (see Table 4). Avoid approaching the extremes because this may cause abnormalities. As a rule it is preferable to rear embryos within the lower ranges of their temperature tolerances, to hold back bacterial growth. A temperature of 10°–18° C. is adequate for most species. If possible, use a constant-temperature room or a refrigerator. Avoid sudden changes in the temperature; let eggs warm up slowly to room temperature before using them. Protect embryos carefully from direct sunlight and from heat from the Bunsen burner and from the lamp on the operating table.

Since the rate of development is temperature-dependent, it is possible to obtain a desired stage of development, at a specified time, by manipulating the temperature. It is also possible to obtain different stages of development from the same cluster by speeding up part of the embryos and slowing down others. The necessary time schedules have to be worked out empirically. For data on rates of development, see page 20.

4. *Selection of material for operations.*—Absolutely normal and healthy material is a prerequisite for successful operations. If a cluster contains numerous dead or abnormal embryos, the normal-looking embryos are often weak; discard the entire cluster if you can afford it, or else separate the normal embryos immediately. Discard all eggs and early embryos that exhibit white spots (disintegrating cells), discharge cells, or show blisters or edema. Discard eggs or embryos that are retarded in their development—as compared with the majority in the same cluster—or show abnormalities, such as microcephaly (abnormally small head) or curvatures in body or tail or irregular outgrowths.

5. *Preparation for operations.*—Prepare in advance a sufficient number of instruments, particularly those made of breakable material, to have a supply on hand in case an instrument breaks during the operation. Prepare the instruments *exactly* according to specifications (pp. 3 ff.). In some instances, it is not possible to give standard specifications, as, for instance, with respect to the tips of glass needles (p. 7). Much time and effort are wasted if glass needles are used that are inadequate for a particular operation or stage. They may be too coarse or too fine, too long (hence too flexible) or too short, too blunt or too pointed. Prepare in advance a set of needles with different points and try them out on the embryo. Ask your laboratory instructor to check your instruments. Sharpen and clean all metal instruments carefully. Use scouring powder for removal of rust.

All instruments and pipettes used for *fixatives* and other chemicals should be kept off the operating table and strictly separated from those used for living material. Mark them with a glass pencil or a gummed label.

Dishes.—Have a number of sterilized dishes with agar bottom and sterile lids on hand. With a sturdy glass needle or ball tip (p. 8) make grooves in the agar immediately before the operation. Have an embryo in the dish and adjust size of groove to size of embryo. To avoid injury to the embryo, be sure that the grooves have smooth edges. If transplantations are done, make two grooves side by side, for donor and host. Fill the operation dish with concentrated medium and place one or two sterile glass bridges in the dish.

6. *Rules for operations.*—All motions in operating and transferring embryos and in lifting dishes that contain embryos should be made slowly and gently. Avoid jerky movements and shaking, particularly of operated gastrulae and neurulae. Handle the embryos as little as possible and work fast but without haste. After an operation allow for sufficient time for healing before transferring the embryo to another dish. Be careful in *pipetting* embryos. Because of the high surface tension of water-air interfaces, naked embryos, or parts which are brought accidentally in contact with the surface, are instantly disrupted and spread over the surface. Therefore avoid air bubbles in the pipette; submerge it before water is sucked in. Fill it with water before embryos or parts are sucked in and, keeping it submerged, pick up the material by gentle release of the rubber cap or membrane (of micropipettes). In transferring, turn the bent tip of the pipette upward and release pressure on rubber cap. Be sure that the mouth of the pipette is submerged well below the surface before you release the contents. Do all pipetting of small embryos and isolates under the binocular microscope. For turning the embryo, use hair loops or platinum loops only.

Observe all *sterilization* measures rigorously. Each student must have within easy reach a small alcohol or Bunsen burner, a coplin jar or a small beaker with 90 per cent alcohol, and a Syracuse dish with sterile culture medium. If possible he should also have a small beaker with boiling water.

Go through the following routine each time you use an instrument:
Dip glass needle in boiling water, or if not available, in alcohol and then in culture medium.
Dip hair loop in alcohol and then in culture medium.
Pull mouth of pipette, glass bridge, ball tip through flame.
Dip metal instruments in alcohol and then hold them over the flame.

Culture medium.—Use *full-strength culture medium* for all operations (unless directed otherwise); leave embryos in full-strength medium until completely healed. *Rear all embryos in dilute medium* and all isolates (explants) in full-strength solutions.

Place each operated embryo in a separate dish, cover it with a lid, and give it a protocol number at once.

43

Always do several operations of the same kind. You have to count on some mortality even if all precautions are taken; also some of your operations may have been unsuccessful.

7. *Postoperative handling.*—Keep operated embryos cool; the temperature in the laboratory should be kept below 20° C. (70° F.). Check operated embryos at least once a day, but otherwise avoid handling and disturbing them. Observe the same precautions of sterility and careful pipetting as under section 6. Keep the dishes covered with a lid. Remove dead embryos at once. Fix valuable operated embryos when they show the first signs of lesions, cell loss, edema, or blisters. Once disintegration starts, it proceeds rapidly. When embryos reach advanced tail-bud stages (around stage 30 in *Ambystoma*), transfer them from agar dishes to dishes without agar bottoms or to paraffined paper cups.

8. *Records.*—Keeping a careful record of each operation is just as important as the operation itself. Give each type of operation a designation—as, for instance, "bal." for balancer transplantations—and give each operated embryo a serial number, such as bal. 1, bal. 2, etc. Label the dish containing the operated embryo, or the lid, with a glass pencil. Prepare a separate sheet for each embryo. The protocols for different operations will differ in detail, but the following data should appear at the head of each sheet: species, type of operation, serial number, date and hour of operation, stage of embryo, and exact description of operations, including a sketch. At least once a day during the days following the operation, record your observations; give as much detail as possible. Sketches are usually very helpful. For a sample protocol see page 88.

After the termination of each experiment, add to your protocol sheets a brief statement indicating the question which the experiment was supposed to answer and the conclusions that can be drawn from your results. Compare your results with those of the other members of the class. Be sure to have a clear understanding of the theoretical implications of each experiment that you perform.

5. CHECK LIST OF STANDARD EQUIPMENT

1. CHECK LIST OF EQUIPMENT FOR EACH STUDENT

Dishes

several 4-inch finger bowls (250 ml.) or large paraffined paper cups to keep eggs or egg masses before operation

several casters (or Syracuse dishes) for decapsulation, etc.

6–12 casters with agar and wax bottoms for operations and for postoperative rearing of young stages (p. 11)

12 glass plates, $2\frac{1}{2}$ sq. in., as lids

Other tools and instruments
low-power dissecting microscope (low power 9 × or 12 ×; high power
18 × or 24 ×)
microscope lamp or gooseneck lamp with heat filter
alcohol lamp for sterilization
beaker, tripod, Bunsen burner, asbestos plate (for boiling water, for sterilization of glass needles, etc.), or Stender dish with alcohol and dish with
dilute medium (for cleaning of glass instruments)
Erlenmeyer flask for concentrated culture medium
Erlenmeyer flask for $\frac{1}{10}$ per cent culture medium
2 pairs of watchmaker forceps
1 pair of ordinary small forceps
1 pair of scissors
1–2 scalpels
6 pipettes of different sizes, including a large-mouthed pipette (5 mm. in
diameter) for transferring of eggs in capsules
rubber caps of corresponding sizes for pipettes
1 micropipette
several glass needles
several hair loops or platinum wire loops
several glass rods with ball tips of different sizes
wooden holder for the 3 last-mentioned items
rack of wire for pipettes
6–12 glass bridges of different sizes in small Petri dish with lid
glass jar laid out with cotton to keep metal instruments in 95 per cent
alcohol

2. CHECK LIST FOR CLASS EQUIPMENT

Equipment
refrigerator, kept at 12°–18° C., for keeping of embryos
glass rods and tubing (soft glass) for preparing glass instruments (see p.
3).
Bunsen burner and microburner (mounted on stage) for preparing glass instruments
files and diamond pencils
fine grain oil stone and oil for sharpening of watchmaker forceps
6–10 crystallizing dishes or $7\frac{1}{2}$-inch finger bowls for egg masses
stock of paraffined paper cups and $2\frac{1}{2}$-sq.-in. lids of glass

Solutions
6-liter flask, stock solution of full-strength Holtfreter or other solution
6-liter flask, 10 per cent Holtfreter or other solution
6-liter flask, boiled tap water or spring or pond water, for eggs in capsules
and swimming larvae

MS 222, 1:6,000 or chloretone, 1:3,000 for narcotization
streptomycin sulfate
penicillin
sulfadiazine
formaldehyde (10 per cent formol) for preservation of whole embryos (for sectioning use Bouin's fluid).

B. DESCRIPTION OF GASTRULATION IN URODELES

An intimate knowledge of the process of gastrulation in amphibians is indispensable for an understanding of the experimental work done on early embryos. During gastrulation the germ layers are formed by extensive cell movements. Moreover, transplantation, explantation, and other experiments have shown that, during and shortly after gastrulation, some of the main organ primordia become more or less rigidly "determined." In other words, profound changes in the visible and invisible organization of the embryo take place during this period. The morphogenetic cell movements are now clearly understood, thanks to the admirable vital-staining experiments of Walther Vogt (1925, 1929) and his collaborators. The following presentation is largely based on their work.

1. THE STRUCTURE OF THE URODELE EMBRYO BEFORE AND AFTER GASTRULATION

The blastula is spherical and clearly polarized. The "animal" hemisphere is characterized by several layers of small cells which form the thin roof of the "blastocoele." They contain little yolk and are usually pigmented. The cells of the "vegetal" hemisphere are heavily laden with yolk and are unpigmented.

At the end of gastrulation, i.e., shortly before the medullary plate makes its appearance, the embryo (Fig. 8) is still spherical in shape, but it has acquired a visible bilateral symmetry, and its walls are formed by three sheets, the germ layers. The blastocoele is almost entirely replaced by another central cavity—the primitive gut or archenteron. The archenteron is actually closed and plugged by the yolk plug up to early neurula stages. It opens to the outside by withdrawal of the plug (Brown, 1941). The ectoderm forms a complete outer covering continuous with the mesoderm around the blastopore. It is usually pigmented throughout; the unpigmented cells have been shifted inside. The mesoderm forms a mantle subjacent to the ectoderm. However, the anterior-ventral part of the embryo remains free of mesoderm, and the mesoderm mantle ends with a free edge, which extends in an oblique direction from dorsal-anterior to ventral-posterior (me in Fig. 5). This sharp edge fades out near the mid-dorsal line, where the anterior-dorsal part of the mesoderm mantle merges with the anterior-dorsal part of the entoderm. The anterior part of the archenteron is the foregut, which is disproportionately wide at this stage. The entoderm behind the foregut forms a troughlike structure partly inside of, and covered by, the mesoderm mantle. Its massive floor is formed by the large, yolk-laden cells. Its anterior and lateral walls are thinner and rise steeply from the floor. The walls do not meet in the mid-dorsal line (at least not in the stage under consideration) but appear as two parallel lines, lateral to the median plane (*e*, in Figs. 7–10). Thus the archenteron has a dorsal gap and no entodermal roof. However, the dorsal part of the mesoderm mantle becomes intimately applied to the free edges of the entodermal trough and thus forms temporarily a lid over the archenteron; for this reason the dorsal part of the mesoderm mantle, at this stage, has been given the misleading name "archenteron roof." In the neurula stage the free entoderm edges will converge and, eventually, fuse underneath the mesodermal mantle, thus giving the archenteron its permanent entodermal roof. The temporary contact of archenteron roof and entoderm is so intimate that cross-sections may simulate an actual fusion. Such pictures were taken as evidence in favor of the entodermal origin of the mesoderm and particularly of the notochord. The investigations of Vogt and of others before him leave no doubt that this conception is erroneous; both germ layers originate at the blastopore and remain separate units, despite their temporary contact.

This latter statement requires a qualification. There is, indeed, true continuity of mesoderm and entoderm at two places: in a narrow, sickle-shaped area ventral to the blastopore and, as mentioned before, in the roof of the headgut. The situation in this latter area is difficult to visualize and deserves further comment. *Ch* in Figure 9 marks the anterior end of the prospective notochord. At this point the mesoderm does not end abruptly, as will the notochord in later stages, but continues into the so-called "prechordal plate." In its cellular texture the prechordal plate appears as a true transitional zone between ento- and mesodermal structures. A sagittal section exactly through the median plane shows, therefore, a continuous archenteron roof partly of entodermal and partly of mesodermal origin. Such sections figure prominently in most textbooks. Yet they are liable to give a wrong conception of the entoderm-mesoderm relation, unless they are presented in conjunction with transverse sections.

2. EXTERNAL FEATURES OF GASTRULATION

The transformation of the blastula into the gastrula is accomplished by a sequence of integrated cell movements. The greater part of the vegetal hemisphere invaginates into the interior around the blastopore. The animal hemisphere spreads and overgrows the vegetal hemisphere and eventually forms the entire surface of the neurula. During this process the blastopore changes its shape continuously. These changes vary in different forms and will be described for *A. maculatum*. In Harrison's stage series only 3 gastrulation stages (H10–H12) are distinguished. This proved to be insufficient for experimental workers. Lehmann (1926) and Boell and Needham (1939) have inserted several intermediate stages. We have adopted the seriation of the latter authors and have added another intermediate stage (H12½). We distinguish the following stages (see Fig. 45a):

Stage

H9. . . . . .blastula
H10. . . . . .early blastopore
H10½. . . . . .sickle-shaped blastopore
H10¾. . . . . .semicircular blastopore (½ moon)
H11. . . . . .horseshoe-shaped blastopore (¾ moon)
H11½. . . . . .large yolk-plug stage
H12. . . . . .small yolk-plug stage
H12½. . . . . .slit-shaped blastopore
H13. . . . . .neural-groove stage

The incipient blastopore appears as an irregular line between the equator and the vegetal pole (stage H10). It assumes the shape of a sickle (stage H10½) and acquires a marked bilateral symmetry. Its plane of symmetry, which coincides with that of the future embryo, only now becomes apparent, although it is "determined" much earlier.[7] The region of the animal pole is the future anterior end of the embryo; the blastopore itself marks the future anal region. The meridian connecting the animal pole with the middle of the blastopore is the future mid-dorsal line. The area above the blastopore is the so-called "upper" or "dorsal lip" of the blastopore. Next, the blastopore begins to elongate and to encircle the yolk field. Its semicircular shape (stage H10¾) indicates that the areas lateral to it begin to invaginate around the "lateral lips." The blastopore then assumes the shape of a horseshoe (stage H11). Eventually, the lateral invagination grooves complete the encirclement of the yolk field, which gradually disappears to the inside (formation of a ventral lip). The exposed part of the yolk in the stage of the circular blastopore is called "yolk plug" (stage H11½). The rapid inward movement of the yolk cells continues, the yolk plug becomes small (stage H12) and eventually disappears entirely. The blastopore has now assumed the shape of a short slit (stage H12½), which extends in longitudinal direction (i.e., perpendicular to the early blastopore) and marks the future anus. This stage is conventionally considered the end of gastrulation. Shortly afterward the medullary plate becomes visible (stage H13). From this stage on up to that of the closed neural tube, the embryo is called a "neurula."

3. W. VOGT'S METHOD OF LOCALIZED VITAL STAINING AND ITS GENERAL RESULTS

Gastrulation is primarily a phenomenon of cell movements and not of cell division and proliferation. Many attempts have been made to study the cell movements, e.g., by inserting a fine glass needle into the blastula wall and fol-

[7] In some species a "gray crescent" appears shortly after fertilization in the region of the future upper lip of the blastopore, and its plane of symmetry already marks that of the embryo.

lowing its shift. This and similar methods are inadequate for several reasons. The most serious objection is that such mechanical devices may interfere with normal development. Decisive progress was made when W. Vogt applied a method of localized vital staining.[8] The procedure is, briefly, as follows: A small particle of agar stained with Nile blue sulfate or neutral red is pressed against the surface of the blastula for a short period. Such marks remain distinct and well circumscribed for several days. According to Vogt, diffusion of the stain into neighboring cell areas is negligible, and the marks do not interfere with normal development. In this way it is possible to follow the movements of the marks throughout gastrulation by continuous observation. Particularly instructive were those experiments in which blastulae or early gastrulae were marked by a series of alternating red and blue marks (as many as fourteen on one embryo) and their shifts relative to each other observed. In an exhaustive analysis Vogt obtained almost complete records of the gastrulation movements of all parts of the surface area, and, eventually, he was in a position to outline a coherent picture of the mechanics of germ-layer formation. The same experiments solved another problem of no less importance. Since the marks persisted over a considerable time, it was possible to establish their ultimate locations in the organ primordia by microdissection of early tailbud stages. This, in turn, enabled Vogt to "project" the pattern of the organs back onto the surface of the blastula or of the early gastrula. His maps of the organ-forming areas of blastulae and early gastrulae are well known. They are an invaluable help not only for a better understanding of gastrulation but as guides in transplantation and other experiments.

The limitations of Vogt's method should be clearly understood. The designations of the different areas on the maps indicate merely their actual fate ("prospective significance," Driesch) in normal, undisturbed development. They do not imply that the early gastrula is built up of discrete mosaic stones, which differ actually from one another in structure or otherwise. Such a view would misinterpret entirely the methodological rank of the vital-staining technique. It is a tool for refined observation of normal development, i.e., a descriptive method, not an analytical method. It does not reveal intrinsic properties or potencies of the stained areas. Only potency tests like transplantation or isolation experiments are suitable for such an analysis. It is correct to refer to the areas on the map as "prospective notochord," etc., but not as "notochord" or "notochord primordium."

4. MAPS OF THE EARLY URODELE GASTRULA

Maps of the early gastrula are reproduced in Figure 4. Similar maps for the urodele blastula and for the anuran gastrula may be found in Vogt (1929) and

[8] Similar methods had been devised previously by Goodale (1911) and Detwiler (1917).

Pasteels (1942). The map requires little comment. Its outstanding landmark is the line (*il*) which separates the invaginating material (prospective ento-derm and mesoderm) from the non-invaginating prospective ectoderm. The prospective mesoderm forms a ring or girdle around the yolk field. It is broad-est on the dorsal side and narrowest on the ventral side. In the German litera-ture it is known as the *Randzone* ("marginal zone"). A peculiar feature of the map should be noted: the areas which will form the axial organs have their greatest extent in a direction perpendicular to the median plane, i.e., perpen-dicular to their ultimate position. Thus the prospective medullary-plate area forms a transverse band with pointed lateral ends; the prospective notochord is a sickle-shaped area above the blastopore; the somites are lined up in two transverse rows, etc. It requires a considerable "wheeling" to maneuver all prospective areas into their ultimate positions.

Vogt's map, which was largely based on experiments on the European *Tri-turus* species, has been revised by Nakamura (1938), using the Japanese newt *Tr. pyrrhogaster*, and by Pasteels (1942), using the *Axolotl* (*A. mexicanum*). The maps of Pasteels are reproduced in Figure 4, *C* and *D*; they apply prob-ably to other *Ambystoma* species as well. Both authors are in virtual agree-ment with each other. Their maps are in all essential points identical with those of Vogt but differ from the latter in several details, as follows:

The shape of the prospective notochord area is different; in particular, its lateral horns are less pointed and do not extend as far lateral as they do in Vogt's map. According to Pasteels, the ventral marginal zone is largely pro-spective lateral-plate material (*l*), whereas Vogt considers the greater part of this area as prospective trunk and tail somite material (*t*). According to Pas-teels, the latter material extends to the median dorsal line and forms a narrow strip between the prospective notochord and medullary plate. Furthermore, Pasteels has made detailed studies of the origin of the different parts of the somites which, on his map, form very long and narrow strips. As was to be expected, that part of the prospective somite region which is adjacent to the prospective notochord material represents the inner, median edges of the fu-ture somites, and the part adjacent to the prospective lateral-plate area (*l*) represents the ventral edges of the somites. The outer, lateral borders of the somites cannot be stained by superficial marks and must therefore be located in the deeper layers of the marginal zone (see p. 56).

5. FORMATION OF THE MESODERM

The mesoderm mantle is formed by an invagination of the mesoderm girdle, or marginal zone, around the blastopore. *Invagination* is one of the four basic gastrulation movements, as distinguished by Vogt. The fact that the blasto-pore makes its first appearance in a dorsal position and gradually encircles the

yolk indicates a definite sequence in time of the invagination of different mesoderm areas. The dorsal mesoderm (prospective notochord) invaginates first;
somite material follows around the lateral lips; eventually the ventral part of
the marginal zone is tucked in. As a general rule, areas which are located nearest to the blastopore will invaginate first, and their final position inside will be
farthest away from the blastopore; material which invaginates late will settle
near the blastopore.

The map shows that the blastopore originates entirely within the yolk field.
Therefore, prospective entoderm will be the first material to invaginate; it will
be carried into the head region and will form there the anterior blind end of the
archenteron, that is, the anterior parts of floor, walls, and roof of the future
pharynx. Accordingly, the gill slits are mapped out on the early gastrula at a
short distance from the early blastopore. The dorsal entoderm is immediately

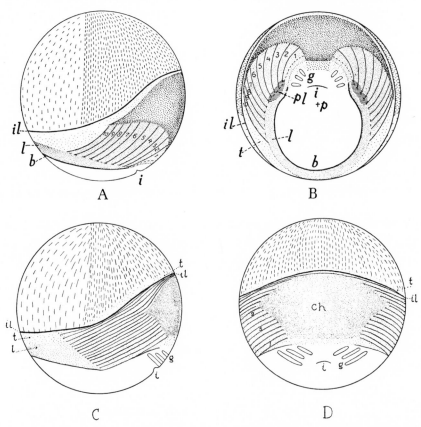

Fig. 4.—Maps of prospective areas of urodele embryos at the beginning of gastrulation. *A*, lateral
view; *B*, dorsal view of *Triturus* (from Child, 1941, after Vogt); *C*, lateral view; *D*, dorsal view of
axolotl (after Pasteels, 1942). Denser broken lines, neural plate; less dense broken lines, general
ectoderm; coarse stippling, notochord; fine stippling, mesoderm; *b*, ventral lip of blastopore; *ch*,
notochord; *g*, gill area; *i*, beginning of invagination; *il*, limit of invagination; *l*, lateral mesoderm;
p, vegetal pole; *pl*, pronephros and forelimb area; *t*, prospective tail region; 1–10, somites 1–10.

52

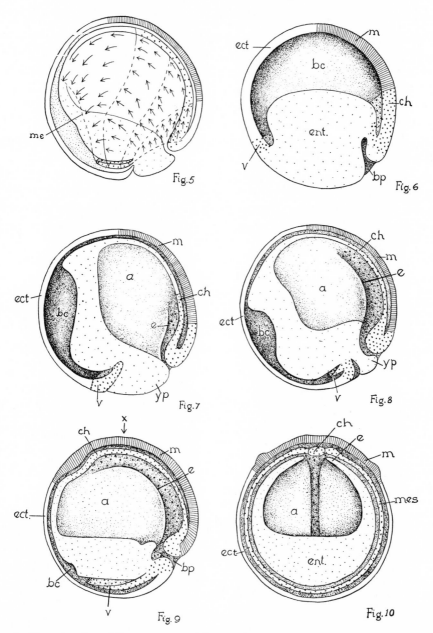

Fig. 5.—Reconstruction of the movements of the mesoderm mantle, projected on a middle gastrula stage (urodele). The dotted lines indicate the anterior edge of the mantle in four different stages. *me* = anterior mesoderm border at the end of gastrulation (Fig. 9). The area anterior to *me* is the "mesoderm-free field." The arrows indicate the directions of movements (after Vogt, 1929).

Figs. 6–10.—Gastrulation in urodeles (reconstruction after diagrams and sections, in Vogt, 1929). Fig. 6, beginning of gastrulation. Fig. 7, large yolk-plug stage. Fig. 8, small yolk-plug stage. Figs. 9–10, early medullary-plate stage. Figs. 6–9, median sections. Fig. 10, transverse section cut in plane *x* of Fig. 9: posterior half of neurula. *a* = archenteron; *bc* = blastocoele; *bp* = blastopore; *ch* = notochord; *e* = upper edge of the entoderm trough; *ect* = ectoderm; *ent* = entoderm; *m* = medullary-plate material; *v* = ventral mesoderm; *yp* = yolk plug.

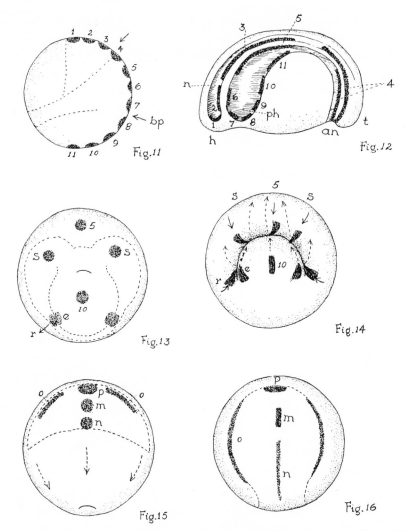

FIGS. 11–16.—Vital-staining experiments on urodele gastrulae (Figs. 11–14, after Vogt, 1929; Figs. 15, 16, after Goerttler, 1925).

FIG. 11.—Eleven marks (*1–11*) placed in the median line of a late blastula. Lateral view. The upper arrow indicates the border of invagination; bp = point of origin of blastopore. The dotted lines indicate the borders between the main prospective areas (see Fig. 4, *A*).

FIG. 12.—The same embryo in early tail-bud stage, with position of marks *1–11*. An = anus; h = head; n = neural tube; ph = pharynx; t = tail.

FIG. 13.—Marking of prospective mesoderm and entoderm in the early gastrula. Ventral view. The dotted lines indicate the borders between prospective areas (see Fig. 4, *B*). Marks *5* (prospective notochord) and *10* (median entoderm) as in Fig. 11; e = mark on outer edge of entoderm field; r = mark on ventrolateral part of marginal zone (prospective lateral mesoderm); s = mark on anterior somite material.

FIG. 14.—The same embryo as in Fig. 13, in middle gastrula stage. Note the changes in shape and in position of the marks. The solid arrows indicate the direction of past movements on the surface; the dotted arrows indicate the movements after invagination. Designations as in Fig. 13.

FIG. 15.—Marking in the prospective medullary-plate area (dotted lines) of the early gastrula stage; m, n = marks in the median line; o = lateral marks; p = mark on the animal pole. The arrows indicate the directions of movements.

FIG. 16.—The same embryo as in Fig. 15, in medullary-plate stage.

followed by the prechordal material, which in turn is followed by the anterior end of the prospective notochord material. This, then, is the first mesodermal area to be tucked under. In order to visualize clearly the fashion in which the notochord material is brought into its final position, let us follow two marks placed on prospective notochord areas. Mark *5* (Figs. 11, 13) is located in the median plane and has a central position in the notochord area. It will move toward the blastopore, invaginate around its dorsal lip, and disappear. While it is still outside, it will change its shape: it will elongate and, at the same time, become slightly narrower; this expansion in the longitudinal direction will continue after its invagination. Eventually, the formerly circular mark will stain a surprisingly long strip of the narrow notochord. Mark *5* (Fig. 12) illustrates well the enormous degree of elongation which the prospective notochordal material undergoes. Almost all parts of the gastrula undergo varying degrees of expansion during gastrulation. *Elongation or expansion* is the second basic gastrulation movement.

A mark placed laterally to mark *5* will move radially toward the blastopore. This area is destined to form the posterior part of the notochord. After it has arrived at the blastopore, it will invaginate and, at the same time, move toward the median plane. The direction of its motion inside is different from its course outside; it "converges" toward the median plane. The lateral wings of the notochord area will undergo an even higher degree of convergence. We shall see that convergence is characteristic not only of lateral notochordal material but of other lateral material as well, be it invaginating or non-invaginating. It is by this directional movement that lateral areas are swung into more median positions. *Convergence* is the third basic gastrulation movement.

The somite material is found on the map in a position lateral (and, according to Pasteels, partly dorsal) to the early blastopore. As is to be expected, the material of the first somites is nearest to the blastopore; it will invaginate first. A mark placed on the prospective anterior somites (Fig. 13, *s*) will move toward the blastopore in an approximately radial direction and will converge perceptibly toward the median line and thus reach its destination near the median axis (Fig. 14). A relatively small circular mark will stain parts of several somites and thus indicate the conspicuous elongation of the material which has taken place. Again, invagination, convergence, and elongation are instrumental in placing somite material in its ultimate position. An unexpected discovery was made when the lateral and ventral lips of the *slit-shaped* blastopore were stained. These areas were found to invaginate as late as in early neurula stages and to form the somites posterior to somites 8–10. This means that, in a stage when gastrulation seems to be completed, not more than about 8 somites have actually invaginated and that invagination of somite (and other mesoderm) material continues for a considerable time and in the same fashion as before, with simultaneous convergence and elongation. Vogt calls this phase the "late invagination" and emphasizes the fact that "the moment of the closure of the blastopore is not a decisive hiatus, neither in the formation of the axial mesoderm nor of the trunk as a whole" (1929, p. 452). However, the invagination of notochord and entoderm are terminated in the slit-shaped blastopore stage, and "late invagination" involves only non-chordal mesoderm.

Unsegmented lateral and ventral mesoderm (hypomere) forms a narrow ring adjacent to the yolk field; it invaginates around the ventral and lateral lips of the blastopore in a very late phase of gastrulation. In the large yolk-plug stage lateral invagination has just begun; in the small yolk-plug stage the ventral mesoderm mantle appears inside as a wedge-shaped structure (v in Fig. 8) which grows out of the ventral and lateral lips of the blastopore and pushes forward between ectoderm and entoderm. The lateral plates are represented on the surface map of the early gastrula as a surprisingly narrow strip (somewhat larger on Pasteels' map), whereas they cover a wide area inside in the neurula and later stages. Notice the rapid progression of the anterior edge of the mesoderm mantle (Fig. 5). Expansion accounts largely for the observed increase in surface; the material becomes thinner while it spreads. However, this is not the complete story. Vogt was puzzled by the observation that certain organs, as, for instance, the heart, were stained only by very deep marks but not by light marks, which would stain merely the superficial cells. Thus he was led to the deduction that the anterior regions of the mesoderm mantle are formed by material which never lies on the surface of the early gastrula but is located in deep layers of the marginal zone. This material he calls the "inner marginal zone." It proceeds forward, forming the anterior edge of the mantle; in moving, it expands and receives reinforcement from behind, first from the stock of "inner marginal zone," piled up in the ventral and lateral blastopore lips and later on from the invagination of superficial, or "outer marginal-zone" material, as described above. The origin of heart, blood islands, head mesoderm, and outer lateral edges of somites (p. 51) from the inner marginal zone is definitely established.

The entire mesoderm mantle, including notochord, somite, and hypomere material invaginates, of course, as a continuous unit. The arrows in Figure 5 indicate the direction of movement at different points of this uniform field. If the dorsal and dorsolateral areas converge toward the dorsal mid-line, as they do, then the ventrolateral and ventral areas must compensate for this movement by increased expansion and by a corresponding movement in dorsal (and anterior) direction. These movements appear as a fanlike, divergent spreading when viewed from the ventral side. Vogt has called this component of the gastrulation movements "divergence." It may be considered as a fourth basic movement, although it is really nothing but a consequence of the convergence of dorsal material. In fact, the divergence of ventral mesoderm appears likewise as a "convergence" toward the dorsal mid-line, when viewed from above.

6. THE FORMATION OF THE ENTODERM AND ITS SEPARATION FROM THE MESODERM

We remember that the blastopore appears within the boundary of the yolk field (prospective entoderm) and that the structures which are the first to invaginate are to form the purely entodermal anterior end of the archenteron, i.e., the pharynx. Marks *7* and *8* (Figs. 11, 12), which are placed in the median line immediately above and below the blastopore, illustrate the situation. The lumen of the head gut swells rapidly and extensively in the first phases of gastrulation, whereby the lumen of the blastocoele becomes obliterated. While the notochord and somite materials follow the head-gut material around the dorsal and lateral lips in true invagination movements, the ventral yolk glides into the interior underneath the arch of the sickle- and horseshoe-shaped blastopore as a continuous stream without actual invagination around a groove; a ventral lip is non-existent during these phases of gastrulation. Vogt once compared this shift with the retraction of a stretched-out tongue. A mark placed in the middle of the yolk field (*10* in Figs. 13 and 14) illustrates this movement. The mark elongates while it approaches the blastopore and disappears under the blastoporal groove. Having arrived inside, it moves forward and will be found eventually as a broad patch in the middle of the floor of the intestine (Fig. 12). It can be shown that all prospective entoderm material which was located in the median line before invagination will form the median floor of the intestine. Obviously, lateral parts of the yolk field will form the lateral walls of the archenteron trough. Mark *e* in Figure 13 likewise moves toward the blastopore and elongates in a direction almost parallel to mark *10*. In its progression inside, it spreads farther and, at the same time, moves upward and converges toward the median plane. It will be found eventually in the upper edge of the left wall of the archenteron. A mark between *10* and *e* would stain an area in the middle of the lateral wall of the archenteron. Again, regions near the blastopore will form anterior parts of the intestine, and regions at a distance from the blastopore will invaginate later and form posterior intestine. The entoderm formation is completed with the disappearance of the yolk plug (Fig. 9), and no "late invagination" of entoderm occurs.

A new problem arises when we visualize mesodermal marginal zone and entodermal yolk field as being continuous on the surface of the blastula but entirely separate structures at the end of gastrulation (except in the pharyngeal and in the blastoporal region). Even their directions of movement inside are divergent: The mesoderm mantle spreads forward and downward, the walls of the entoderm move upward. Their separation must occur sometime during gastrulation. According to an earlier view, which was widely accepted for a long time, this would happen by invagination of a uniform "archenteron" and subsequent delamination of the mesoderm from the entoderm. The mesoderm would be a derivative of the entoderm, i.e., of "gastral" origin. According to an alternative interpretation, the separation takes place before or during invagination, and the two germ layers invaginate as autonomous units: "peristomial" origin of the mesoderm. It is one of the outstanding contributions of Vogt to a theory of gastrulation to have established for urodeles the correctness of the second alternative. If one considers for a moment marks e and r (Fig. 13) as one single mark, then one finds that this mark is cut in two at the moment when it arrives at the blastoporal groove (Fig. 14). From then on, the two parts take entirely different courses (see arrows), and eventually are widely separated—one in the lateral plate, the other at the upper edge of the entodermal trough. Marks which are partly on entodermal and partly on mesodermal territory were actually studied, and the reality of the rupture was demonstrated beyond doubt. Accordingly, the horseshoe-shaped line on the map (heavy in Fig. 4, B, and stippled in Fig. 13) designates more than the border line between entoderm and mesoderm; it demarcates the line of rupture; and its absence (on the map) between prospective gills and first somites merely expresses the fact that entoderm and mesoderm remain continuous in the pharyngeal region.

7. THE GASTRULATION MOVEMENTS OF THE PROSPECTIVE ECTODERM

The gastrulation movements of the prospective ectoderm (Figs. 15 and 16) were studied by Vogt's collaborator, K. Goerttler (1925), and by Schechtman (1932, for *Taricha torosa*). Since the embryo retains its size and its spherical shape throughout gastrulation, the animal hemisphere (prospective ectoderm) must be expected to compensate for the invaginating ventral hemisphere by extensive expansion and thinning. This is demonstrated by every mark placed on the prospective ectoderm, except on the animal pole. The extent and direction of the movements of different parts of the ectoderm will be discussed separately for prospective epidermis and prospective medullary plate.

Prospective medullary plate.—If the animal pole is stained (Fig. 15, p), then the mark will be found, first, in the anterior, transverse part of the medullary fold, and later on in the floor of the forebrain. Its shape is almost unaltered. The animal pole, then, is the only area of the gastrula which remains stationary. Marks placed in the median line will stay in the mid-line and elongate in the direction toward the blastopore. The nearer to the blastopore, i.e., the nearer to the future posterior end, the more will a mark elongate during gastrulation and neurulation (compare m and n). The median marks will be found in the floor of the spinal cord. It is important to notice that all material which is located in the median line of the early gastrula remains there and thus makes true "concrescence" (i.e., "growing together") of lateral areas impossible. The lateral parts converge toward the median line, but never concresce. The same was stated before for the notochord. (True concrescence takes place when the neural folds fuse or in heart development, but nowhere in gastrulation.) Lateral marks show clearly the convergence of the lateral parts of the prospective medullary material. Mark *o* in Figure 15 is particularly suitable to illustrate the "wheeling" movement (*Schwenkung*, Goerttler) toward the median line, the fixed point being the median end of the mark near the animal pole. The parts of the mark which are farthest away from the midline traverse the longest distance. This wheeling movement takes place largely during the first part of gastrulation; it is followed by elongation during the later phases of gastrulation.

The prospective *epidermis* occupies the ventral sector of the animal hemisphere. Its movements are in conformity with those of the prospective medullary material. They are characterized by a very considerable expansion in a fanlike fashion. In ventral view this expansion appears as a "divergence." The old term "epiboly" ("growing over") may well be applied to this maneuver, since this spreading is, at the same time, a process of growing over the invaginating mesoderm and entoderm.

8. SUMMARY

The prospective medullary area and the prospective notochord have several features in common. Their longest diameter is in a transverse direction before gastrulation and in longitudinal direction afterward. The gastrulation movements of their median, as well as of their lateral, parts are almost identical, although the one invaginates and the other does not. Their movements are perfectly integrated with each other, since they have a long border in common along which they remain continuous throughout gastrulation. A similar comparison may be drawn between the divergence of ventral and ventrolateral ectoderm and that of ventral and ventrolateral mesoderm. All these observations taken together illustrate emphatically the integration of all gastrulation movements, the uniformity of the process as a whole, whose basic trends— elongation, convergence, divergence, etc.—transcend the border lines of invaginating and non-invaginating areas and of the prospective germ layers.

BIBLIOGRAPHY

BOELL, E. J., and NEEDHAM, J. 1939. Morphogenesis and metabolism: studies with the Cartesian diver ultramicromanometer. III. Respiratory rate of the regions of the amphibian gastrula. Proc. Roy. Soc. London, B, **127**:363.

BROWN, M. G. 1941. Collapse of the archenteron in embryos of *Amblystoma* and *Rana*. Jour. Exper. Zool., **88**:95.

DETWILER, R. S. 1917. On the use of Nile blue sulfate in embryonic tissue transplantation. Anat. Rec., **13**:493.

GOERTTLER, K. 1925. Die Formbildung der Medullaranlage bei Urodelen. Arch f. Entw'mech., **106**:503.

GOODALE, H. D. 1911. The early development of *Spelerpes bilineatus*. Amer. Jour. Anat., **12**:173.

LEHMANN, F. E. 1926. Entwicklungsstörungen in der Medullaranlage von Triton, erzeugt durch Unterlagerungs-Defekte. Arch. f. Entw'mech., **108**:243.

NAKAMURA, O. 1938. Tail formation in the urodele. Zool. Mag., Tokyo, **50**:442.

PASTEELS, J. 1942. New observations concerning the maps of presumptive areas of the young amphibian gastrula (*Amblystoma* and *Discoglossus*). Jour. Exper. Zool., **89**:255.

SCHECHTMAN, A. M. 1932. Movement and localization of the presumptive epidermis in *Triturus torosus* Rathke. Univ. of Calif. Pub. in Zoöl., **36**:325.

VOGT, W. 1925. Gestaltungsanalyse am Amphibienkeim mit örtlicher Vitalfärbung. I. Methodik. Arch. f. Entw'mech., **106**:542.

———. 1929. Gestaltungsanalyse am Amphibienkeim mit örtlicher Vitalfärbung. II. Gastrulation und Mesodermbildung bei Urodelen und Anuren. *Ibid.*, **120**:384.

C. EXPERIMENTS

1. PROSPECTIVE SIGNIFICANCE OF EMBRYONIC AREAS (VITAL STAINING)

a) PREPARATION OF DYED AGAR

Nile blue sulfate and neutral red are generally used as "vital" (that is, non-toxic) dyes. They are applied by means of an agar carrier (read p. 49 f. for general orientation). Usually, the dyed agar is prepared in two steps. Prepare a 1–2 per cent solution of agar (c.p.; powder or shreds) in distilled water and boil briefly until the agar is completely dissolved. Stir with a glass rod. While the solution is still warm, pour thin films of agar on a set of carefully cleaned microscope slides or larger glass plates. Allow the agar to dry thoroughly (several days); protect the slides from dust. Next, prepare a 1 per cent solution of Nile blue sulfate and a 1 per cent solution of neutral red (preferably from Gruebler), in distilled water. Do not use culture medium, because the dyes precipitate in salt solutions. Dissolve the dyes completely—if necessary by gentle heating. Pour the dye solutions in large Syracuse dishes or other dishes and submerge the agar plates in this solution. Cover the dishes and let them stand for several days. Wash off excess dye and allow the agar to dry again in a dust-free place. The agar plate is then ready for use or for storage in a sterile wrapping. One can prepare the dyed-agar plate in one step by adding the dye to the agar solution before it is poured on the glass plates.

When you are ready for the experiment, moisten a small area of the agar with a drop of water. Allow the agar to soak up the water (several minutes) and scrape off small chips with a (sterile) scalpel. Place small pieces in the operation dish or a Syracuse dish and, under the binocular microscope, cut out small square pieces of suitable size, using scissors or a fine steel knife. Do not use too small pieces for your first experiments. Let the pieces of agar stand for a few minutes until clouds of stain are no longer given off. The success of marking experiments depends largely on a strong concentration of the dye in the agar. Use only deeply stained agar plates.

b) VITAL-STAINING EXPERIMENTS ON THE EARLY
GASTRULA OF URODELES

Read carefully Section B (p. 47); consult the maps of prospective areas on Figure 4, page 52. The vital-staining experiments are "experiments" only in the sense that they involve manipulation of the embryo. They do not interfere with the normal developmental processes, however, and they do not reveal causal relationships. They are not "analytical" experiments, differing in this respect from most of the other experiments dealt with in the following sections of this *Manual*. They merely make visible certain aspects of the normal developmental processes that are otherwise hidden to direct observation because of the absence of natural markings.

Material for Experiments 1–3
> *Ambystoma,* any species; *Diemictylus*
> *Taricha torosa,* particularly suitable because unpigmented
> stage H10 to H10$\frac{3}{4}$
> agar, dyed with neutral red or Nile blue sulfate
> standard equipment (p. 44)
> operation dishes with wax bottoms (preferable to agar bottoms)

EXPERIMENT 1: STAINING OF THE UPPER LIP OF THE BLASTOPORE (FIG. 17)

Procedure

1. Select a number of healthy gastrulae. Remove the outer capsules, but leave the vitelline membrane intact, for the time being. Wash the embryos in sterile dilute culture medium.

2. Prepare the operation dish. Fill it with warm water, which softens the wax bottom layer. Make several grooves of suitable size with the ball tip. The size of the groove is important; it has to fit the gastrula snugly and should cover at least the lower hemisphere. It is advisable to sacrifice one gastrula for the purpose of exact fitting. Smooth the edges carefully. Replace the water with culture medium. Place several glass bridges in the dish.

3. Place a drop of culture medium on the dyed-agar plate (choose one which is intensely impregnated with dye). After 1–2 minutes, when the agar has taken up water, scrape off small chips of agar with a scalpel or steel knife, transfer a piece of these scrapings to a Syracuse dish, allow excess dye to diffuse out, and cut out a square piece, of adequate size to cover the upper blastoporal lip. It is advisable for beginners to use rather large pieces. Transfer several agar pieces to the operation dish.

4. Place a gastrula in the groove. You will observe that the embryo rotates and comes to rest in a position with the animal pole upward and the blastopore not in sight. To reduce the tendency to rotate, and to facilitate staining, it is advisable to puncture the vitelline membrane and release the perivitelline fluid. Puncture the vitelline membrane several times near the animal pole with a fine glass needle or tear a very small hole in the vitelline membrane with 2 pairs of very finely sharpened forceps (p. 9) but do not remove the membrane altogether. The dye diffuses through the membrane. Try to avoid injury to the embryo.

5. Gently lift the embryo with hair loops and turn the blastoporal region upward. While it rotates back slowly, mark the position of the blastopore on the edge of the groove. After the embryo has come to rest, push a piece of dyed agar between it and the wall of the groove, at the previously marked point (Fig. 17). If necessary, trim the agar piece further. If the agar piece is not tightly applied to the surface of the embryo, it is advisable to weigh the embryo down with a glass bridge.

5a. If the groove fits very tightly, you may be able to orient the embryo in a position with the blastopore facing upward. In this case, the orientation of the dye mark can be made more precise. Place the agar piece on top of the gastrula, over the middle of the upper blastoporal region and press it against the embryo with a glass bridge. It may be necessary to weigh down the glass bridge with small pieces of glass cut from microscope slides. Watch for back-sliding of the bridge.

6. Allow 20–45 minutes for staining, depending on the concentration of the

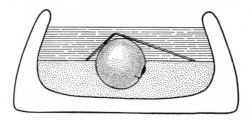

FIG. 17.—Vital staining of early gastrula (see text)

dye in the agar. The mark should be deeply red or blue. Gently lift the embryo out of the groove and transfer it to an agar dish with *dilute* culture medium.

7. In this experiment it is particularly important to have a very accurate sketch of the position and extent of the mark; the interpretation of the results depends on it. In experiments done according to 5 (rather than 5a), the mark may not be exactly in the middle of the upper blastoporal lip. This does not matter, since variations in the position of the mark will give interesting information on the fate of different areas of the dorsal marginal zone (prospective mesoderm).

8. During the next 24 hours make frequent observations and sketches of the invagination of the stained area (but handle the embryo as little and as gently as possible). Observe the gradual stretching of the mark, and its convergence, if the mark was lateral. Note the change in the shape of the blastospore. The medullary-plate stage is of particular interest, since the stained notochord is usually visible under the medullary plate, demonstrating vividly the enormous stretching and narrowing which the originally square area has undergone.

9. Terminate the experiment in an early tail-bud stage. Carefully dissect the embryo, either alive or after a short (3–5 minute) fixation in 10 per cent

formaldehyde. (The dye will fade out when fixation is prolonged.) Mount the embryo in a groove, dorsal side up. Very cautiously remove the dorsal epidermis and the neural tube with a rather strong glass needle, thus exposing notochord and somites. Indicate on a sketch precisely the extent of the stained area and compare with the original sketch. This gives a projection of the stained structure onto the surface of the early gastrula (Vogt's mapping), and the intervening sketches give an idea of the cell movements which have brought the structure to its final position.

Note.—Make 3 or 4 experiments of the same type.

Experiment 2: Vital Staining of Prospective Somites

Stain an area of the upper blastoporal lip distinctly to the left or to the right of the median plane. Proceed as before.

Experiment 3: Vital Staining of the Prospective Medullary Plate

Place a mark between the blastopore and the animal pole, nearer to the latter (Figs. 15 and 16). During the following days note the elongation of the stained material. If the mark was not in the mid-line, note its convergence toward the median plane.

Further suggestions—Stain other parts of the early gastrula—for instance, in the region of the future lateral or ventral blastoporal lip. Stain the animal pole and note that the mark scarcely changes its position and shape. Where is it located in the early tail-bud stage? After having acquired some experience, try to place two marks on the embryo and note the shifting of the marks with respect to each other. (Vogt succeeded in placing as many as 17 marks on one embryo!)

c) Vital-Staining Experiments in the Neurula

Material for Experiments 4–6
    same as for Experiments 1–3; stages H14 and H15

Experiment 4: Vital Staining of the Prospective Eye-forming Area
(Manchot, 1929; Woerdeman, 1929)

Procedure
    Remove all membranes, including the vitelline membrane. Place a mark on the anterior median part of the medullary plate. The mark should cover the slope of the transverse medullary fold, in stage H15 (Fig. 26). Allow the embryo to develop to stage H26 or H29. The stain on the eyes will be visible from the outside. Fix the embryo in 10 per cent formaldehyde. Shortly after fixation

carefully dissect the head in an operation dish with wax bottom. Remove the epidermis with a glass needle and slit the brain open at the dorsal side. Determine the extent of the stained area in the brain and the eyes. If the original mark extended too far posterior, then the floor of the forebrain and midbrain may be found stained. It is surprising to find that the area in the early medullary plate from which both eyes originate is one uniform, median region, not separated by a piece of prospective brain. During neurulation the mark will gradually expand to the sides and become dumbbell-shaped. The lateral parts will be folded up and come to lie in the lateral walls of the forebrain, from where they are evaginated as optic vesicles. The narrow median part of the mark will persist in the optic stalks. The part of the brain that separates the eyes in later stages is derived from material that was located posterior to the eye area in the early medullary plate and has moved forward during neurulation. These findings have been of great importance in the interpretation of the origin of cyclopia, a malformation in which one single median eye, instead of two eyes, is found (see Adelmann, 1936).

EXPERIMENT 5: VITAL STAINING OF THE PROSPECTIVE NASAL, BALANCER, LENS, GILL, EAR ECTODERM
(Carpenter, 1937)

Procedure

Remove the jelly membranes but not the vitelline membrane. Mount the neurula in a depression in an operation dish so that the prospective head region points upward. Stain one of the areas listed above, using Figure 18 for your orientation. Make several experiments. Follow the shifting of the marks during neurulation and make sketches of transitional stages and of the position of the mark in stages H29–H35. Dissect the head, if necessary.

EXPERIMENT 6: VITAL STAINING OF THE BORDER BETWEEN HEAD AND TRUNK

Procedure

Place a mark on the mid-line of the medullary plate, slightly posterior to the mid-point of the anterior-posterior axis, where the folds come closest together, or place the mark on a corresponding point outside the right medullary fold (*B* in Fig. 18). Raise the embryo to stage H24 or older. Locate the mark; dissect if necessary. Count the number of somites in front of the mark. This experiment is very informative in that it demonstrates a point which is not always realized, namely, that the anterior two-thirds of the neurula represent the head and anterior part of the trunk and that the greater part of the trunk and the tail are telescoped in the posterior third of the neurula. The posterior end, and particularly the tail bud, stretch very extensively in subsequent stages.

65

Aquatic vertebrates, including amphibian larvae, possess a special type of sense organs, the lateral-line organs, which are receptors for water pressure and aid the animal in its orientation in flowing water. They are cup-shaped structured composed of sensory and supporting cells and are exposed to the surface. They are arranged in lines that form specific patterns on the head,

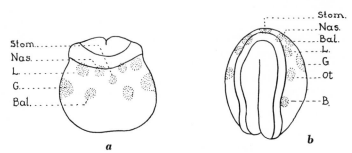

FIG. 18.—Vital staining of head structures of urodele neurulae (after Carpenter, 1937). *B* = border between head and trunk; *Bal.* = balancer; *G* = gills; *L* = lens; *Nas.* = nasal placode; *ot.* = otocyst; *Stom.* = stomodeum.

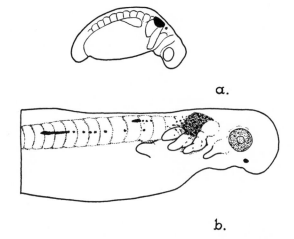

FIG. 19.—Vital staining of the lateral-line placodes (from Stone, 1933). (See text.)

trunk, and tail. Those of the head are innervated by a special branch of the facial nerve; those of the trunk and tail by a branch of the vagus nerve.

Their mode of origin is unique in several ways. The three trunk and tail lines characteristic for urodele larvae originate from ectodermal thickenings, or "placodes," which are located immediately behind the otocyst. The deeper cells of these placodes become detached and migrate caudad in a body. They glide along the inner surface of the epidermis in three distinct columns, forming one dorsal, one middle, and one ventral line. On their way they deposit, at regular intervals, clusters of cells which differentiate into the cup-shaped sense organs. The latter push through the ectoderm and are thus exposed to the surface. All placode material is used up when the migrating primordia have reached the caudal end of the tail. The primordium of the sense organs is accompanied by the lateral-line branch of the vagus nerve, which originated at about the same time and in a fashion similar to that of the sense organs, i.e., from a vagus placode. Side branches of this nerve innervate each individual sense organ. The lateral-line organs of the head and their nerves originate in a similar fashion from placodes in front of the otocyst (see Stone, 1922, 1933).

The mode of origin of the lateral-line sense organs is of particular interest because it demonstrates long-range directional migration of cell groups along specific paths. This process can be observed on the living embryo with the aid of vital staining. The intriguing problem of the determination of the lateral-line pathways has instigated a classical experiment of Harrison (1904), in which parts of darkly pigmented embryos of *R. sylvatica* were combined with parts of the lighter *R. palustris* embryo and the deposition of dark sense organs on the light epidermis was observed. This was one of the first instances in which the method of heteroplastic transplantation (previously worked out by G. Born) was applied in an analytical experiment. Stone has continued this analysis, using the methods of transplantation of placode primordia and of vital staining. His papers (1922, and particularly 1933) should be consulted.

EXPERIMENT 7

Material
    same as for Experiments 1–3, stages H28–H30
    the unpigmented embryos of *Taricha torosa* are particularly suitable
    dyed agar plates
    standard equipment (p. 44)
    MS 222 for narcosis

Procedure
    1. Select healthy tail-bud stages, not younger than stage H28. Remove all membranes.
    2. Make a rather shallow depression in the operation dish, to fit an embryo lying on its side. Transfer several glass bridges to the operation dish and place the embryo in the depression, right side up.
    3. Locate the otocyst above the second visceral arch. Place a medium-sized piece of deeply stained agar over the area immediately posterior to the otocyst and dorsal to the gill swelling (Fig. 19, *a*). Hold the agar in position with a glass bridge. Press tightly. Stain for 15–30 minutes, or more if necessary. Be sure to get a deep stain of the epidermis.
    4. After removal of the glass bridge, make a sketch of the head, indicating

accurately the stained area. Transfer the embryo to a glass dish or small paraffined paper cup.

5. Observe the embryo twice a day, for several days, under the high power of the binocular dissecting microscope, using the best light source that is available. The ordinary laboratory lamp (p. 3) is inadequate. Observe the rather rapid lengthening of the median line extending across the middle of the somites. It is an elongated, club-shaped structure that moves in caudal direction and leaves behind on its path darkly stained spots, the lateral-line sense organs. The primordium of the dorsal line starts somewhat later and lengthens in the same fashion. It turns dorsad and follows the upper border of the somites (see Fig. 19, *b,* and Stone, 1922, Figs. 1–12; also Stone, 1933, Figs. 1–3). Make careful sketches.

Further suggestion.—Stain a corresponding area directly in front of the otocyst and study the formation of the lateral line system of the head.

BIBLIOGRAPHY

ADELMANN, H. B. 1936. The problem of Cyclopia. Quart. Rev. Biol., **11**:161–284.

CARPENTER, E. 1937. The head pattern in *Amblystoma* studied by vital staining and transplantation methods. Jour. Exper. Zool., **75**:103.

HARRISON, R. G. 1904. Experimentelle Untersuchungen über die Entwicklung der Sinnesorgane der Seitenlinie bei Amphibien. Arch. Mikr. Anat., **63**:35.

MANCHOT, E. 1929. Abgrenzung des Augenmaterials und anderer Teilbezirke in der Medullarplatte. Arch. f. Entw'mech., **116**:689.

STONE, L. S. 1922. Experiments on the development of the cranial ganglia and the lateral-line sense organs in *Amblystoma punctatum*. Jour. Exper. Zool., **35**:421.

———. 1933. The development of lateral-line sense organs in amphibians observed in living and vital-stained preparations. Jour. Comp. Neurol., **57**:507.

WOERDEMAN, M. W. 1929. Experimentelle Untersuchungen über Lage und Bau der augenbildenden Bezirke in der Medullarplatte beim Axolotl. Arch. f. Entw'mech. **116**:220.

2. SOME ANALYTICAL EXPERIMENTS IN PREGASTRULA STAGES

a) ARTIFICIAL PARTHENOGENESIS IN THE FROG

Fertilization, that is, the union of the two gametes, has two important consequences. By the fusion of egg and sperm nuclei, the diploid chromosome number is restored and two different sets of nuclear hereditary factors are combined. Furthermore, fertilization activates the first cleavage and thus initiates development.

The occurrence of parthenogenesis (i.e., development of the egg without insemination) in a number of animals—for instance, in rotifers, aphids, *Cladocera,* and the honeybee—shows that neither the fusion of two cells nor the fusion of two nuclei is a prerequisite for the initiation of development. In 1901 Jacques Loeb made the discovery that the sea-urchin egg can be stimulated to develop into a normal larva without fertilization by placing it in hypertonic sea water ("artificial parthenogenesis"). The conclusions drawn from normally parthenogenetic eggs can thus be extended to eggs which normally require the sperm for activation. Many different chemical and physical agents are now known to activate eggs: for instance, surface-active substances like fatty acids, which have a slightly cytolyzing effect; hypertonic and hypotonic salt solutions; temperature changes; irradiation; and pricking with a fine needle. In addition to the sea-urchin and starfish eggs, those of several annelids; of mollusks; of the frog, the rabbit, and others have responded to such treatments. Students who are interested in the theories that have been advanced to account for the activating role of the sperm on the basis of artificial parthenogenesis experiments are referred to the reviews by Tyler (1941, 1955). See also Wilson (1925) and Morgan (1927).

Artificial parthenogenesis in the frog's egg.—The frog's egg is rather refractory to chemical agents; but in 1910 Bataillon discovered that artificial parthenogenesis may be obtained by puncturing the egg with a fine needle of glass or platinum. This treatment is successful, however, only if the needle is dipped into frog's blood and a small amount of blood is introduced into the egg. Shaver (1953) found that cell-free extracts of different adult frog and mammalian tissues are equally effective and that the activating agent is associated with cytoplasmic particles (mitochondria and microsomes). The role which this agent plays in activating the egg is not known, but its indispensability has been confirmed by all observers.

A small percentage of parthenogenetic frogs develop into tadpoles, and Loeb, Parmenter, and others have succeeded in raising a number of these through metamorphosis to sexual maturity (see photographs in Loeb, 1921). The chromosome situation in these specimens is of particular interest. Parmenter (1933, 1940) found a number of young tadpoles to be haploid; but all those which had metamorphosed were diploid. According to Parmenter, the regulation of the chromosome number may occur before cleavage starts. It will be remembered that the frog's egg is in the stage of the second maturation spindle when insemination takes place. In cases of experimental parthenogenesis the spindle may be withdrawn into the egg and the formation of the second polar body suppressed, so that the egg starts with a diploid number of chromosomes (all derived from the female pronucleus). Or both polar bodies may be formed, but the first nuclear division may not be followed by a cytoplasmic division and the two chromosome sets reunite.

EXPERIMENT 8

Material

2 ovulating females of *R. pipiens* or other frog species (experimental ovulation; see p. 28)

see p. 28

69

1 non-ovulating female as a source of blood
3–4 clean microscope slides per student
pipettes
Petri dishes or finger bowls
1 Syracuse dish
3–4 fine, *straight* glass needles
scissors, scalpel or tissue lifter
paper towels
spring or pond water or dilute culture medium

Sterilization.—In this experiment it is imperative that contamination with sperm be avoided. Sterilize all glassware and instruments, and remove all male frogs from the laboratory.

Procedure

1. Prepare the blood of the non-ovulating female as follows: Wash the female and pith it. Open the abdomen and expose the heart. Cut off the tip of the ventricle and let the blood accumulate in the pericardial cavity or in the coelom. Close the abdominal skin flaps until ready to use the blood.

2. Strip the eggs of the ovulating female on sterile slides (see p. 31). Place 2 rows of eggs on each slide. Prepare 3–4 slides in this way.

3. Dissect a leg muscle of the frog which has been bled, dip it in the blood pool in the abdominal cavity, and smear all eggs with blood. Avoid exerting pressure on the eggs.

4. Dip the tip of the glass needle in the blood surrounding the egg and, under good illumination, puncture each egg at some point in the animal hemisphere. Avoid injury to the germinal vesicle, which is usually located directly at the animal pole. Be sure that the tip of the needle has entered the egg and that blood corpuscles have been introduced with the needle. The puncturing of the cortex results in the outflow of some egg material (exovate) which should not be extensive. Leave the eggs on one slide untreated, as controls, and mark them as such.

5. As soon as a slide has been finished, immerse it in sperm-sterile spring or pond water or dilute culture medium in a Petri dish or small finger bowl. Indicate the time of puncturing in your record.

6. After 10–20 minutes, when the jelly membranes are swollen, separate the eggs gently from the glass by means of a sterile scalpel or tissue lifter. Keep experimental and control material strictly separate.

7. Observe the first cleavage which is to be expected $2\frac{1}{2}$–$2\frac{3}{4}$ hours after puncturing (at 18°–20° C.). Keep the eggs under continued observation for several hours. Notice normal and abnormal cleavage patterns and make sketches of both.

8. After 6–8 hours, calculate the percentage of cleaving eggs. Discard all non-cleaving eggs,

9. Many eggs will stop their development during cleavage and then disintegrate. Remove them at once. Isolate blastulae and gastrulae in individual dishes or small paper cups and follow their development. Compare parthenogenetic with normal tadpoles.

Note.—The percentage of cleaving eggs is highly variable (5 per cent to nearly 50 per cent, in our class experiments); the percentage of eggs that reach gastrulation and later stages is always low. Calculate the percentages for your own material and include in your record the corresponding data for the entire class.

BIBLIOGRAPHY

BATAILLON, E. 1910. Le problème de la fécondation circonscrite par l'imprégnation sans amphimixie et la parthenogénèse traumatique. Arch. zool. expér. et gén., **46**:102.

LOEB, J. 1921. Further observations on the production of parthenogenetic frogs. Jour. Gen. Physiol., **3**:539.

MORGAN, T. H. 1927. Experimental embryology, chap. xxiii. New York: Columbia University Press.

PARMENTER, C. L. 1933. Haploid, diploid, triploid, and tetraploid chromosome numbers, and their origin in parthenogenetically developed larvae and frogs of *Rana pipiens* and *Rana palustris*. Jour. Exper. Zool., **66**:409.

———. 1940. Chromosome numbers in *Rana fusca* parthenogenetically developed from eggs with known polar body and cleavage histories. Jour. Morphol., **66**:241.

SHAVER, J. R. 1953. Studies on the initiation of cleavage in the frog egg. Jour. Exper. Zool., **122**:169.

TYLER, A. 1941. Artificial parthenogenesis. Biol. Rev., **16**:291.

———. 1955. Gametogenesis, fertilization and parthenogenesis. In WILLIER, WEISS, and HAMBURGER (eds.), Analysis of development. Philadelphia: W. B. Saunders.

WILSON, E. B. 1925. The cell in development and heredity, chap. v. New York: Macmillan.

b) ANDROGENETIC HAPLOIDY IN THE FROG[9]

The problem of the role of the nucleus in development has many facets; one of them concerns the effect of quantitative changes in chromosome sets. For higher animals in which all tissue cells, except the gametes, are diploid, the question has been raised whether a single set of chromosomes (haploidy) can support normal development (see Fankhauser, 1945, 1955; Briggs and King, 1959).

Several methods are available for obtaining haploid embryos, one of which, experimental parthenogenesis, was presented in the preceding experiment. In this instance, the egg develops with its own nucleus (gynogenetic haploidy). The experiment to be dealt with below describes a method whereby the egg, deprived of its own nucleus, develops under the direction of the sperm nucleus (androgenetic haploidy). This method, apart from yielding a higher percentage of haploid tail-bud stages than parthenogenesis, has attained particular significance for the analysis of the role of the nucleus through its combination

[9] I am greatly indebted to Dr. R. Briggs for his help in preparing this outline.

71

with the hybridization method. Fertilizing the egg cytoplasm of one species with the sperm of another creates a unique situation which permits evaluation of the respective role of each component in a very direct way. Androgenetic haploid hybrids have been produced in sea urchins and amphibians. The haploid amphibian embryos do not live long enough to show species differences; but this difficulty has been overcome, at least for some structures, by the ingenious device of transplanting pieces of hybrid gastrulae, while they are still in a healthy condition, to normal gastrulae, which serve as their "nurses," the transplants carrying on beyond the life span of the donor gastrulae. Extensive work on urodele hybrids has been done in Switzerland by Baltzer and Hadorn (reviews in Baltzer, 1940, 1952; Hadorn, 1961) and on anurans by J. Moore, Briggs, and others (see J. Moore, 1955; Briggs and King, 1959).

The technique of enucleation of the egg has become of importance in another context. Briggs and King have succeeded in implanting diploid nuclei from blastulae and gastrulae into such enucleated eggs with the intention of testing the potentialities of nuclei from differentiating tissues. They have found that nuclei from blastulae can fully substitute for the zygote nucleus and support normal development but that this capacity decreases in later stages, indicating a progressive differentiation of nuclei (Briggs and King, 1953, 1959).

In the present context, we are concerned only with the question of the developmental capacity of the androgenetic haploid frog embryos and with the technique of enucleation developed by Porter (1939).

The haploids develop normally, though somewhat retarded, through gastrulation. The first structural abnormalities become apparent during neurulation, on the third day. The neural plate is shorter, and the neural folds are less prominent than in the controls. In the following days a characteristic combination of abnormal features becomes manifest; this has been referred to as the "haploid syndrome": The embryo remains shorter than the controls, the head is disproportionately small (microcephaly), the abdomen is swollen and rounded, and gill development and circulation are usually poor. From the seventh day on, an edematous condition develops (tissue spaces filled with fluid) that rapidly becomes more extreme and eventually lethal. Few embryos live longer than 8–10 days (for detailed description see Porter, 1939). Obviously, the haploid nucleus is not capable of supporting development beyond the hatching stage. Several suggestions have been made to account for its insufficiency. For instance, lethal or sublethal recessive genes, not masked by their dominant alleles, have been made responsible. However, this possibility has been ruled out on theoretical grounds and by experiment. It is more likely that the quantitative disproportion of nucleus and cytoplasm accounts for the failure of normal development. It has been suggested that the relatively small nucleus is unable to produce sufficient amounts of enzymes for the utilization of yolk or for other metabolic and synthetic processes. The observation that egg fragments and small eggs produce better haploid larvae than do large eggs speaks in favor of this line of thought (see discussions in Fankhauser, 1955; Moore, 1955; Briggs and King, 1959).

The Swiss school has used Curry's technique of enucleation by sucking off the egg nucleus with a micropipette (Curry, 1931). We present in the following the glass-needle technique of Porter (1939), which is widely used in this country.

EXPERIMENT 9

Note.—This experiment requires special optical outfit and special illumination; it is therefore not suitable as a class experiment. It is suggested that it be used as a demonstration by the instructor or as an assignment for individual students.

Material

ovulating females (hypophysis-injected) and males of *Rana pipiens* or other anuran species

standard equipment for fertilization (p. 29) and operations; finger bowls, paraffined paper cups

microscope slides or watch glasses

pipettes

glass needles, specially prepared. They must be straight, with a very fine, pointed tip, yet stiff and not elastic near the tip. Try different sizes, and prepare 3 or more of suitable size in order to have them on hand if one breaks during the operation.

Optical equipment.—A magnification of 40 × to 60 × is required.

Illumination.—A stronger light source than that recommended for this course is needed. Nicholas illuminator with the front lens removed may be used. The best illuminator for this purpose is the A0 universal microscope light No. 353, fitted with heat absorbing glass disc No. 308. Place it 4–6 cm. from the object, focus to maximum brilliance, and run it at maximum voltage.

Procedure (Porter, 1939; Briggs and King, 1953; Briggs, personal communication)

1. Strip approximately 30 eggs from a female on a clean microscope slide or watch glass (see p. 31).

2. Add sufficient sperm solution to wet the eggs. Place the slide or watch glass in a covered Petri dish.

3. After 5–10 minutes add dilute medium or pond or spring water. The eggs should remain stuck to the glass.

4. Place the eggs at once under the binocular and watch for the appearance of a tiny *black dot* directly at the animal pole. This is the second maturation

73

spindle that has to be removed. It becomes visible about 10–25 minutes after insemination as the result of a dispersal of the pigment granules above the spindle. Focus the light source on the animal pole and search for the black dot in one egg after another. The black dot is very small but distinct (see Briggs and King, 1953, Fig. 4).

5. *Enucleation.*—As soon as you have spotted the black dot, insert the glass needle diagonally through jelly membranes, vitelline membrane, and surface coat of the egg, slightly to one side of the dot. Move the tip of the needle straight up through the dot, making a small tear in the surface coat. A small amount of white material, which should contain the egg nucleus, flows out. With some practice and a sufficiently fine needle, one succeeds in making only a slight injury that does not interfere with normal development. Repeat the experiment on all the eggs in which you can spot the black dot.

Note.—The black dot is visible for only about 15 minutes, whereupon it fades out, signaling the completion of the second maturation division.

6. Strip one or two more batches of eggs and repeat the experiment until you have 20–30 enucleated eggs. Make sham operations on an equal number of eggs, by making exovates at some distance from the animal pole.

7. Carefully remove all eggs from the glass plates and place all enucleated eggs in one finger bowl or Lily cup, and the sham-operated eggs in another. Avoid crowding. Fertilize 20–30 eggs of the same female and keep them as controls. Mark all 3 containers.

8. Observe the cleavage in all groups. During the following days observe the embryos carefully. The first symptoms of haploidy become visible during neurulation. Compare the enucleated and the normal embryos by placing them side by side under the binocular; look for the "haploid syndrome," which is described above and, in more detail, by Porter (1939), and consult his illustrations. In those operated embryos that appear to be entirely normal, the egg nucleus was probably missed, and the egg remained diploid.

9. The typical symptoms, including edema, are clear evidence of haploidy. However, there may be doubtful cases, and an independent check of ploidy is desirable. A simple method for determining chromosome number, the "tail-tip" method, was developed by Fankhauser. The tail tip of a swimming larva, when the tail fins have become transparent, is clipped, stained *in toto* in Harris' acid hemalum, and mounted without sectioning. The technique is described in Fankhauser (1945, p. 22). The size of melanophores and of epidermis cells is also a good indicator of the chromosome number.

A note on polyploidy.—The development of amphibian embryos with 3, 4, or more sets of chromosomes has been studied by a number of investigators, particularly Fankhauser and his co-workers. These investigations were greatly facilitated when effective methods of producing triploidy (by cold and heat treatment of eggs immediately after fertilization) were discovered. The many interesting problems and observations relating to polyploidy are reviewed in detail in Fankhauser 1945 (see also 1955); J. Moore, 1955; Briggs and King, 1959. It is suggested that students interested in this topic work out the experimental procedure of producing polyploid embryos by consulting Fankhauser's review and the original literature.

BIBLIOGRAPHY

BALTZER, F. 1940. Über erbliche letale Entwicklung und Austauschbarkeit. Naturw., **28**:177.
——. 1952. The behaviour of nuclei and cytoplasm in amphibian interspecific crosses. Symp. Soc. Exper. Biol., **6**:230.
BRIGGS, R., and KING, T. J. 1953. Factors affecting the transplantability of nuclei of frog embryonic cells. Jour. Exper. Zool., **122**:485.
——. 1959. Nucleocytoplasmic interactions in eggs and embryos. In BRACHET and MIRSKY (ed.), The cell. New York: Academic Press.
CURRY, H. A. 1931. Methode zur Entfernung des Eikerns bei normal-befruchteten und bastard-befruchteten Triton-Eiern durch Anstich. Rev. suisse de zool., **38**:401.
FANKHAUSER, G. 1945. The effects of changes in chromosome number on amphibian development. Quart. Rev. Biol., **20**:20.
——. 1955. The role of nucleus and cytoplasm. In WILLIER, WEISS, and HAMBURGER (eds.), Analysis of development. Philadelphia: W. B. Saunders.
HADORN, E. 1961. Developmental genetics and lethal factors. New York: Wiley.
MOORE, J. 1955. Abnormal combinations of nuclear and cytoplasmic systems in frogs and toads. Adv. in Genetics, **7**:139.
PORTER, K. R. 1939. Androgenetic development of the egg of *Rana pipiens*. Biol. Bull., **77**:233.

c) ALTERATION OF THE CLEAVAGE PLANE BY PRESSURE

For centuries two alternative theories of development had been under consideration: the *preformation,* or *mosaic,* theory, according to which the organs are preformed in the egg as distinct, though invisible, units, the egg representing a mosaic of these precursors, which merely unfold and grow in the course of development; and the *epigenetic* theory, according to which the egg possesses little, if any, structural diversity, the organs and structures coming into existence gradually, step by step, through interactions of parts and other devices. This basic issue in embryology remained in a controversial state as long as speculation and observation of normal development were the only avenues of approach. When, toward the end of the last century, the powerful experimental method was first applied to the egg and early embryo, the pioneers of experimental embryology, W. Roux, H. Driesch, and others, directed their efforts immediately to an experimental analysis of this problem. Their classical experiments of killing or isolating one blastomere of the 2-cell stage revealed the developmental capacity of a half-egg. According to the mosaic theory, it should form a half-embryo. Since in many instances regulation to a whole embryo took place, the preformation theory in the strict sense was refuted and the way paved for an epigenetic theory (see p. 78).

Further incentive for an experimental test of the preformation theory was given by A. Weismann's "Theory of the germ plasm" (1892). This theory was the first to attribute a decisive role in organ and tissue differentiation to nuclear factors located in the chromosomes; they were designated as "determinants" and are somewhat equivalent to our genes. The cytoplasm was considered merely as building material, which would differentiate under the direction of the determinants. The zygote nucleus was thought to contain a complete assortment of determinants, one set for each organ or tissue. Weismann construed an ingenious scheme whereby the determinants would be segregated and distributed over the different areas of the embryo. The mitotic divisions were considered to be the instruments of segregation: Each cleavage and subsequent division was considered to be a "qualitatively unequal" division, as a result of which the daughter cells would obtain qualitatively different assortments of determinants. For instance, in eggs in which the first cleavage plane coincides with the median plane of the future organism, one blastomere would obtain all determinants for "left" organs, and the other all determinants for "right" organs; the next mitotic division would segregate left-anterior from left-posterior and right-anterior from right-posterior determinants, and so forth, until each cell or tissue type would be left with one type of determinants, which would then be instrumental in the cytoplasmic differentiation of the cell. This theory is the prototype of a preformistic theory; it is a refined nuclear preformation theory. The theory in its original form is untenable, since there is evidence now that in mitotic divisions the daughter nuclei receive qualitatively identical material; but essential elements of the theory are incorporated in the present gene theory of heredity. Recently, Briggs and King (see 1959) have revived the old issue of qualitative differences in the nuclei of different cell types; they have shown in a series of elegant experiments that nuclear differences actually arise in the course of development (though probably as a result not of differential nuclear divisions but of influences of their changing cytoplasmic milieu).

The following experiment of "cleavage under pressure" was one of the first to demonstrate the equivalence of the nuclei in early cleavage stages, thus refuting Weismann's theory for this phase of development. It was first performed by Driesch (1892) on the sea-urchin egg and then repeated successfully on the frog's egg by G. Born (1893) and O. Hertwig (1893). In the sea-urchin egg and in the frog's egg the first two cleavage planes are meridional, but the third is equatorial. If the eggs are mounted on a glass plate, animal pole upward, and then gently compressed by placing another glass plate on top of them, the third cleavage plane will also be meridional. If the pressure is released at the 8-cell stage, the fourth cleavage plane will be horizontal. This procedure does not change the arrangement of the cytoplasmic structure, but it results in a complete reshuffling of the nuclei (see Weiss, 1939, Fig. 33).

Some nuclei that in normal development would be located in dorsal organs now find themselves in a ventral position and, according to Weismann, should determine dorsal structures at the wrong place. Generally speaking, a disorganized patchwork of structures should result if the hypothesis of unequal nuclear division were correct. Instead, normal embryos develop, which proves that the blastomere nuclei cannot be qualitatively different. On the other hand, the experiment gives no clue as to *cytoplasmic* preformation, because the organization of the cytoplasm was not altered.

EXPERIMENT 10

Material
    fertilized eggs of *Rana pipiens* or
       other species
    scalpel
    10 microscope slides per student
    molding clay (permoplast)
    finger bowls
    paraffined paper cups
    glass pencil

Procedure

1. Obtain fertilized eggs by artificial insemination (p. 28).

2. Clean and dry 10 microscope slides thoroughly. Place narrow strips of molding clay near both ends of 5 slides, parallel to the short edges. The strips should not be much higher than the diameter of the eggs in the jelly membranes.

3. About 1 hour after insemination, when the jelly membranes are swollen, cut out 50–60 eggs with scalpel and forceps. Leave them in all membranes. Be sure to select fertilized eggs, whose dark poles face upward. Eggs whose vegetal (light) poles face lateral or upward are usually not fertilized. On each of the slides with molding-clay strips place 10–12 eggs, at some distance apart, each in a small drop of water. Allow time for the eggs to assume their normal position, animal pole upward. Set 10–15 eggs from the same batch aside as controls

4. Place a second slide over the eggs so that the slides are held together by the molding clay. Press the ends slowly but firmly with your thumbs until the eggs are flattened. Check the flattening under the binocular microscope.

5. Watch the appearance of the first cleavage, about $2\frac{1}{2}$ hours after fertilization (at room temperature). The second cleavage follows about 20–30 minutes later. (The times for other amphibians are different.)

6. Observe the appearance and plane of the crucial third cleavage. Mark with a glass pencil all those eggs in which all 3 cleavage planes are perpendic-

77

ular to the glass plates. Make sketches of several of these atypical 8-cell stages and compare them with a normal 8-cell stage.

7. When all eggs on a slide have reached the 8-cell stage, release the pressure cautiously; lift the upper slide by pushing 2 pointed instruments through the molding-clay strips. Discard injured eggs and place all those in which all 8 blastomeres are in one plane in a finger bowl or paper cup. By turning the eggs sidewise, ascertain under the binocular scope that no horizontal cleavage plane is present.

8. Label the dishes and take a record, as follows:

PRESSURE EXPERIMENT

March 22   1:00 P.M. fertilized
             2:00 P.M. 60 eggs compressed
             3:20 P.M. first cleavage in 45 eggs
             4:00 P.M. third cleavage plane meridional in 38 eggs; abnormal in 7

9. One-half to 1 hour later observe the appearance of the first horizontal cleavage plane that is thus delayed by one cleavage step.

10. On the following days make observations on the further development of compressed eggs. Those that develop normally are of crucial importance for our problem. Make sketches of a few embryos. State clearly the results and conclusions in your own words.

BIBLIOGRAPHY

Born, G. 1893. Über Druckversuche an Frosch-Eiern. Anat. Anz., **8**:609.

Briggs, R., and King, T. J. 1959. Nucleocytoplasmic interactions. In Brachet and Mirsky (eds.), The cell. New York: Academic Press.

Driesch, H. 1892. Experimentelle Veränderung des Typus der Furchung und ihre Folgen. Zeitschr. f. wiss. Zool., **55**:1.

Hertwig, O. 1893. Über den Wert der ersten Furchungszellen für die Organbildung des Embryo. Arch. f. mikr. Anat., **42**:662.

Huxley, J. S., and De Beer, G. R. 1934. The elements of experimental embryology, pp. 83 ff. New York: Macmillan.

Morgan, T. H. 1927. Experimental embryology, pp. 473 ff. New York: Columbia University Press.

Roux, W. 1888. Über die künstliche Hervorbringung halber Embryonen durch Zerstörung einer der beiden Furchungszellen. Virchows Archiv., **114**:113. Also: Gesammelte Abhandlungen, **2**:419.

Weismann, A. 1892. Das Keimplasma: eine Theorie der Vererbung. Jena: G. Fischer.

———. 1893. The germ plasm. English trans. New York: Scribner's.

Weiss, P. 1939. Principles of development, pp. 198 ff. New York: Holt.

d) THE PRODUCTION OF TWIN EMBRYOS AND OF DUPLICATIONS IN URODELES

BY CONSTRICTION

Few experiments have influenced the course of experimental embryology more deeply than Driesch's experiment on the sea-urchin egg, in which 2 embryos were produced out of 1 egg by isolating the first 2 blastomeres. This experiment demonstrated an unexpected regulative property in early developmental stages of an organism that shows little regenerative power in adult life. This result was at once interpreted as a strong argument against any preformistic theory of development (see p. 75). It was reasoned that if one half-egg can give rise to a whole embryo, then organ precursors cannot be rigidly fixed in the egg. In regulatory development, the fate of each part of the egg fragment is different from its normal fate, and the normal end result is achieved by adjustments and interactions of the parts, in an epigenetic fashion. Our modern epigenetic theory of development has its roots in this classical experiment. Because of its fundamental importance, it was repeated on the eggs of many other invertebrates and vertebrates, in many instances with the same result.

In the urodele, twin embryos and duplications can be obtained best by constricting the 2-cell stage in the plane of the first cleavage, using a baby's hair (Spemann, 1901, 1902, 1903, 1938; Fankhauser, 1948). Spemann's papers give an exhaustive analysis of the results. When the 2 blastomeres were separated completely by a deep constriction, then the following results were obtained: In a certain percentage of cases 2 whole embryos, that is, "identical twins," developed. They were small in size but otherwise normal. In a larger percentage only 1 blastomere gave a normal embryo, whereas the other half remained an unorganized, though viable, spherical structure. The explanation is as follows: In the first case the first cleavage plane (plane of constriction) coincided with the future median plane of the embryo. In the second instance the first cleavage plane separated future dorsal from future ventral structures, and only the dorsal half gave a normal embryo. The sphere with no axial organs was called "belly piece" (*Bauchstück*). This implies that, in the salamander, the first cleavage plane and the median plane of the embryo have no constant relation. That this explanation is correct can be demonstrated by examining constricted eggs during gastrulation. In some eggs both isolated blastomeres shared in the blastopore and underwent gastrulation, and these eggs invariably gave rise to identical twins. In the majority of cases only one half-egg formed a dorsal lip and gastrulated, and it was this half that developed into the complete embryo, the other forming a belly piece. Spemann concluded that as early as the 2-cell stage the dorsal half differs from the ventral half in that it contains some property which enables it to undergo typical gastrulation and differentiation. This "dorsal quality," which is lacking in the ventral half, was identified later as the "organizer"; and the constriction experiment may thus be considered as the first step in its discovery.

When the two blastomeres are not separated entirely but constricted slightly so that they form a dumbbell-shaped structure, anterior duplication, "duplicitas anterior," may result (Spemann, 1903), resembling the two-headed monsters found occasionally in many vertebrates. The degree of duplication depends on the degree of constriction: slight constriction results in a slight duplication of the head, and such cases may even have a median eye in common; deep constriction, almost to the point of separation, results in embryos that are fused together only at their tail ends. Strangely enough, "duplicitas posterior" (monsters with one head and two posterior ends) never occurred in this experiment. Spemann explains this fact on the basis of the mechanics of gastrulation in constricted eggs (see Spemann, 1938, p. 159). Thus the constriction experiment contributes materially to an understanding of the origin of identical twins and anterior duplications.

In some, but not all, cases of complete and incomplete twinning, the symmetry relations of the internal organs (curvature of the heart and of the intestine, position of liver, gall bladder, etc.) of one twin were found to be inverted. This condition is known as "situs inversus viscerum." The same abnormality is found occasionally in vertebrates. This abnormality is very rare in identical twins in man, but it is the rule in laterally conjoined human twins (Newman, 1940). It is significant that in the constriction experiments all left embryos showed normal situs and right embryos showed the mirror imaging. The experiment of constriction thus broaches another important problem: that of the origin of bilateral asymmetry in vertebrates.

EXPERIMENT 11[10]

Material

Diemictylus viridescens[11] or   hair loop
    Tr. pyrrhogaster   glass dish without agar bottom
2 watchmaker forceps   tap water
baby's hair

Procedure

1. Prepare the hair for constriction.[12] Select a fine hair; hold it between the thumb and forefinger of your left hand so that it forms a loop as indicated in Figure 20, a. Use the natural bend if it is curly. Under the binocular microscope or loupe tie the upper end through the loop twice, using the watchmaker forceps. Then pull on both ends until the diameter of the loop is slightly larger than the smaller diameter of the oval capsule (2–2½ mm. in the case of *D. viridescens*). Cut both ends at some distance from the loop and submerge the loop in the operation dish (without agar bottom).

2. *Prepare the embryo.*—*D. viridescens* females caught in the field during

---

[10] I am indebted to Dr. G. Fankhauser for details of the technique.

[11] *D. viridescens* is preferable because in *Tr. pyrrhogaster* the vitelline membrane frequently bursts under the inner pressure of the constricted capsule, resulting usually in the loss of one half (see Streett, 1940).

[12] Very fine platinum wire may also be used for constriction.

March and April will lay their eggs in captivity. The eggs are folded between the leaves of water plants (see p. 17). The first cleavage occurs 8–10 hours after fertilization. Eggs should be collected twice a day and watched at short intervals, unless the laying has been observed. The outer sticky membrane is milky. In some eggs it can be peeled off, at least in part, and the egg is then visible inside the transparent capsule. If the outer membrane is difficult to remove, leave it intact.

3. *Constriction.*—Wait until the 2-cell stage is well under way. Hold the hair loop upright directly in the center of the visual field so that it appears as one streak. Hold it in place with one forceps and push the egg into the loop with the other forceps (Fig. 20, *b*). When the loop is approximately around

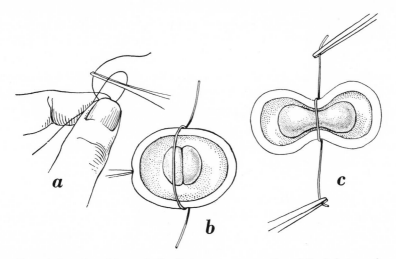

Fig. 20.—Constriction of urodele egg in 2-cell stage. *a* = preparation of the hair loop; *b* = orienting the egg in the loop; *c* = constricting.

the middle of the egg capsule, pull gently at its free ends so that it fits loosely but does not yet constrict. Shift the loop until it is exactly in the middle of the capsule. The slightest asymmetry will result in a conspicuous size difference of the egg halves after constriction, which will obscure the results. Constrict the capsule slightly so that the egg is still free to move in the capsular fluid. Again control the symmetry of the half-capsules; start anew if the halves are unequal. Tilt the egg from one side to the other until the first cleavage plane is exactly under the loop. Then pull slowly and evenly on both ends of the hair until the desired degree of constriction is reached (Fig. 20, *c*). It is sometimes advisable to interrupt the process several times, once the egg has assumed a dumbbell shape. At intervals of 2–5 minutes, the loop is tightened slightly. This procedure lessens the danger of bursting the vitelline membrane.

In order to obtain *complete twins,* it is not necessary to constrict until the two halves are entirely separated. Such a deep constriction usually results in the bursting of the vitelline membrane and the loss of one or both halves. If the bridge between the halves is narrow, it will break apart by itself after a few hours. In order to obtain conjoined anterior duplications, constrict only slightly.

Note.—The same results may be obtained by constricting in one of the planes of the 4-cell stage.

4. After constriction is finished, cut off the free ends of the loop near the egg. Make a sketch, indicating the degree of constriction (diameter of "handle" in proportion to diameter of the lateral halves).

5. Place the egg in a clean dish, in spring or pond water or dilute medium.

6. Observe the gastrulation. It is indicative of the future result. Twins will be obtained if the blastopore and upper lip are shared by both sides. If you find gastrulation in one half only, then you may conclude that the plane of constriction was frontal. The half which does not gastrulate will form a belly piece.

7. Observe further development and make sketches. In the late tail-bud stages the twins will be crowded in the narrow capsule and thus endangered. Try to grasp the hair loop with your sharpest forceps, clip it close to the loop, and remove it. In later stages, when the capsule has lost its turgor, it can be removed easily. However, it is dangerous to do this in early tail-bud stages because the embryos are liable to be squeezed to pieces when the highly turgid capsule is punctured. If whole mounts of the constricted egg with the hair loop intact are desired, fix the egg within the capsules in 10 per cent formaldehyde.

8. Try to raise twins or duplications to stage H40 or older. Observe the situs viscerum of the twins (see p. 80).

BIBLIOGRAPHY

FANKHAUSER, G. 1948. The organization of the amphibian egg during fertilization and cleavage. Annals N.Y. Acad. Sci., **49**:684.
NEWMAN, H. H. 1940. The question of mirror imaging in human one-egg twins. Human Biol., **12**:21.
SPEMANN, H. 1901. Entwicklungsphysiologische Studien am Triton-Ei. I. Arch. f. Entw'mech., **12**:224.
————. 1902. Entwicklungsphysiologische Studien am Triton-Ei. II. *Ibid.*, **15**:448.
————. 1903. Entwicklungsphysiologische Studien am Triton-Ei. III. *Ibid.*, **16**:551.
————. 1938. Embryonic development and induction. New Haven: Yale University Press.
STREETT, J. C., JR. 1940. Experiments on the organization of the unsegmented egg of *Triturus pyrrhogaster*. Jour. Exper. Zool., **85**:383.

3. TRANSPLANTATION EXPERIMENTS TO DEMONSTRATE "SELF-DIFFERENTIATION"

a) INTRODUCTORY REMARKS: TERMINOLOGY

Our epigenetic concept of embryonic development implies that the organ primordia are not yet preformed in the egg but come into existence by gradual "progressive differentiation." The isolation experiments of the first 2 blastomeres (p. 78) gave the first evidence that the different areas of the egg are not yet determined for their fate, since one cell of the 2-cell stage can give rise to a whole embryo. In the terminology of Driesch, the "prospective potency" of the first blastomere is greater than its "prospective significance" (actual fate in normal development). The analysis of the process of organ *determination,* whereby the different areas gradually acquire their specification, has been one of the central issues in experimental embryology. This process became accessible to experimental analysis through the refinement and ingenious application of the method of *embryonic transplantation* by Harrison, Spemann, and a few others. One of the first questions to be answered was that of the *time* of determination of a given organ. It was reasoned that if a small part of an early embryo is transplanted to an atypical position before it is irreversibly determined, then it should differentiate in conformity with its new environment. If transplanted after its destiny is fixed, then it should proceed with its typical differentiation, irrespective of its position in the embryo. By performing this experiment at different stages of development, it should be possible to establish the approximate time at which determination occurs. In his classical transplantation experiments of urodele gastrulae, Spemann (1918) found that if small parts of the "prospective" medullary-plate region and of the prospective epidermis region are interchanged in the *early* gastrula, then the transplants conform to their new position: prospective medullary plate differentiates into epidermis, and prospective epidermis into nerve tissue. If the experiment is done in the late gastrula or early neurula, then prospective medullary-plate material differentiates into nervous tissue, irrespective of its position. These results permit two conclusions: the prospective epidermal and neural regions are relatively indifferent and plastic at the early gastrula stage and acquire their specification during gastrulation, and, furthermore, factors residing in the environment of the transplant, that is, "extrinsic" to it, are responsible for this specification. It was found in later experiments that the subjacent mesoderm mantle is instrumental in the determination of the medullary plate.

Similar experiments of *heterotopic transplantation* (i.e., transplantation to an abnormal position) of prospective limb, balancer, gill, and other regions of the neurula or early tail-bud stage to the flank of another embryo result likewise in the typical differentiation of these organs; they develop as if they had been left in their normal place. W. Roux coined the term "self-differentiation" for this capacity. It implies that the transplants, at the stage of transplantation, contain within themselves all factors essential for their further differentiation, and that they have emancipated themselves from environmental factors. One may properly call these self-differentiating units: limb, balancer, or gill *primordia,* although they are not yet visibly different from one another.

The terms "self-differentiation" and "determination" must be qualified precisely, whenever they are used; otherwise they are misleading and ambiguous.

First of all, it is necessary to identify the *stage* of development for which the self-differentiation capacity of a primordium is claimed. The eyes are self-differentiating in the early neurula, but not earlier. Furthermore, it is necessary to state what specific structural features are to be tested with respect to their self-differentiation or dependent differentiation, because a primordium may be self-differentiating in one aspect of its development but, at the same time, dependent on extrinsic factors in other aspects of its differentiation. For instance, in the early tail-bud stage of a salamander a certain area in the flank will differentiate into a forelimb when transplanted heterotopically; it is self-differentiating from that stage on, as far as its general morphogenesis is concerned. However, experiments of Harrison have shown that the same primordium, at the same stage, is not yet irreversibly determined with respect to its "laterality"; this primordium may develop into a right or a left fore limb, depending on the site of implantation. It still depends on extrinsic factors for its symmetry relations. In Experiments 13 and 14 the following question will be raised: Is the balancer primordium, which is self-differentiating as a whole from tail-bud stages on, dependent on, or independent of, its adjacent structures with respect to the direction of its outgrowth and the time of its resorption? Likewise, the central nervous system is blocked out roughly in the medullary-plate stage; it will differentiate into nervous tissue and even into special parts (forebrain, spinal cord, etc.) when transplanted heterotopically. However, many structural details are not yet determined at that stage but become fixed in later stages under the influence of factors extrinsic to the nervous system. For instance, the size of the spinal ganglia is controlled by the developing peripheral structures to be innervated; the extirpation of a limb primordium results in a size reduction of the limb-innervating ganglia. In this respect the nervous system is not self-differentiating but remains under extrinsic control up to a late stage of differentiation. In other words, determination is not a single act but a process of gradual emancipation from extrinsic factors. Many other instances of the relativity of self-differentiation will be illustrated in the following experiments.

In the analysis of the process of determination the following three questions are pertinent:

1. At what stage of development does a given embryonic area become relatively self-differentiating, that is, independent of certain extrinsic factors?

2. Which components of the developmental processes (e.g., morphogenesis of the whole organ, its symmetry relation, its quantitative growth) are self-differentiating at a given stage?

3. With respect to what extrinsic structures or factors (e.g., adjacent tissue, innervation, hormones) is the primordium under discussion independent or dependent?

The following experiments illustrate relative self-differentiation of whole-organ primordia. They are designed to stress these points: (1) to acquaint the student with the method of transplantation, (2) to illustrate the fact that in the neurula and tail-bud stages of amphibians many organ-forming areas are self-differentiating units as far as their gross morphological differentiation is concerned, and (3) to impress the student with the fact that the process of determination involves changes in the invisible properties of embryonic materials. The primordia to be transplanted are in no way distinguishable from adjacent areas, yet they behave differently in transplantation experiments.

The balancer primordium was found to be a particularly favorable object for the first exercise in transplantation. It is easy to locate and easy to handle. The transplant shows visible differentiation two days after operation, and no dissection or sectioning is necessary for its identification. Furthermore, the balancer offers an excellent opportunity for the study of interesting side issues. For instance, the question of whether the direction of its outgrowth is determined by intrinsic factors or by the surrounding host tissue may be analyzed by varying the orientation of the transplant. Likewise, the question of whether the time of its resorption is determined by intrinsic factors or by the host may be studied by using hosts and donors of different ages.

b) TRANSPLANTATION OF BALANCERS IN URODELES

"The balancers are a pair of slender rod-like appendages which project from the side of the head a little behind and below the eyes, and which . . . serve as props to hold the head off the bottom and to prevent the larva from falling over to its side, until the forelegs develop and assume that office" (Harrison, 1924, p. 349).

They are characterized by a club-shaped thickening at their ends, which secretes a sticky mucus. This "secretion cone" and its stickiness should be used as a criterion for the identification of transplants as "balancers." Transplants which do not show it may be rudimentary balancers or merely epidermal outgrowths. Stickiness can be tested easily with a hair loop. The balancer is innervated by a fine nerve and vascularized by a small artery and a small vein. Its rigidity is maintained by the firm "basement membrane," which is located at the base of the epithelium.

In *A. maculatum* the balancers become visible externally in stage H34; they begin to secrete mucus in stage H38 and reach their full size in stages H40 or H41. The balancers are transitory larval organs that have only a short life span. In *A. maculatum* regressive changes (constriction at the base) begin at stage H45; soon afterward the entire balancer is shed by breaking off at the base. In *A. opacum* the balancer disappears in a different fashion. It shrivels, beginning at the tip, and is largely resorbed. The remnant seems to be cast off as in other forms. Balancers are found only in certain species of urodeles, for instance, in most species of *Triturus*, in *A. maculatum*, *jeffersonianum*, *opacum*, and *microstomum* but not in *tigrinum* (except for a few local strains, in which rudimentary balancers were described by Nicholas, 1924).

Students should study the structure, development, and disappearance of normal balancers before starting experimental work. Harrison (1924) should be consulted for all details concerning their development and histological structure, and Kollros (1940) for details concerning their disappearance.

The experiment is supposed to demonstrate the self-differentiation of the balancer primordium after it is determined but before it is visible. Harrison (1924) has found that, when prospective balancer ectoderm in stages H28 or younger is transplanted to the head of another embryo, it will form a balancer, but, when transplanted to the flank, it will not do so. The same ectoderm taken from stages older than H28 will grow out to form a balancer in any region. Harrison concluded that up to stage H28 prospective balancer epidermis is not entirely self-differentiating but is still dependent on the underlying head mesoderm. Therefore it is advisable always to include the underlying mesoderm in the transplant.

EXPERIMENT 12

Material
    Ambystoma maculatum or *opacum* (*A. tigrinum* has no balancers), in stages
       H27–H31
    standard equipment (p. 44)

Procedure (see also p. 41 and Fig. 21)
    1. Select two embryos of approximately the same stage; remove all membranes, including the vitelline membrane (see p. 37). Fill the operation dish with *full-strength* culture medium.

    2. Transfer both embryos in a wide-mouthed pipette to the operation dish (Syracuse dish with smooth agar bottom). Dip the pipette under the surface of the water before releasing the embryo.

    3. With a glass rod with ball tip make two grooves, one beside the other, of such size and shape that the embryos fit into them snugly when lying right side up. Carefully smooth the edges. Place the embryos in the grooves, right side up. Place several glass bridges of appropriate size near the embryos.

    General rule.—Operate on the right side only; use the left side as a control.

    4. *Prepare the host embryo.*—As the site of implantation choose either the anterior trunk region immediately below somites 6–8 (behind the pronephros) or the region immediately behind, or in front of, the otocyst (Fig. 21, *b*). Avoid the flank and belly region because implants do not "take" well in the yolky material. The first step is the preparation of a cavity to hold the transplant.

This groove should be smaller than the transplant, so that it is held tightly by the surrounding tissue. Make a slit in the epidermis in the following way: Pierce the epidermis at the lower end of the projected cavity with the point of the needle; then push the needle gently forward underneath the epidermis and pierce it again at the upper end of the future cavity, as if you were making a stitch in sewing (Fig. 21, a). Stroke the hair loop gently against the epidermis along the needle until the epidermis is cut. It will retract to both sides. Remove some of the underlying mesoderm. The final preparation of the groove can wait until the transplant is ready for implantation.

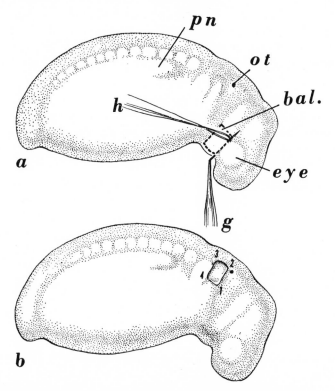

Fig. 21.—Balancer transplantation. a = donor embryo; glass needle (g) and hair loop (h) in the position in which they are held during the operation. The needle is pushed forward under the epidermis. bal. = balancer forming area; ot = otocyst; pn = pronephros region. b = host embryo; 1–2–3–4 = groove prepared for implantation of the transplant.

5. *Extirpate the prospective balancer region in the donor embryo* (*bal.* in Fig. 21, a).—This region is located immediately posterior and adjacent to the eye, on the mandibular arch. Its dorsal border is level with the dorsal border of the eye; its ventral border is above the mid-ventral line and parallel to it. The anterior limit is along the posterior margin of the eye, and its posterior limit is the groove which separates the mandibular arch from the second arch. Very cautiously cut these four edges with glass needle and hair loop, as

described under 4. Start with the anterior edge, then cut the posterior edge, then the ventral line (cut in or slightly above the ventral mid-line), and finally the dorsal line. Carefully avoid disturbing and loosening the underlying mesoderm. After the rectangular piece of epidermis is completely isolated, cut out a substantial pad of the underlying mesoderm, which must remain attached to the epidermis. Very gently lift out the transplant and transfer it with the tip of the needle or with the hair loop near the host embryo and deposit it temporarily on the agar near the implantation site. The beginner is advised to make the transplant rather large; material may get lost in transfer or during implantation. In transferring, try to retain the proper orientation of the transplant; do not rotate it.

Note.—To assure implantation in the right orientation, it is advisable to place a vital-stain mark on the right upper corner of the transplant before it is extirpated (see p. 61).

6. *Implantation.*—If necessary, enlarge the cavity in the host embryo by gently pulling apart the edges and removing more mesoderm cells with the tip of the needle. With hair loop or glass needle lift the transplant into the groove and gently press it down until its epidermal covering is flush with that of the host. The better the edges of host and transplant epidermis are in apposition to each other, the better are the chances of a successful "take." Sometimes one can make the edges fit with the tip of the glass needle. Place a glass bridge over the transplant. It should cover the entire transplant and hold it firmly in position. Be sure to use a glass bridge of the proper size. Work cautiously but fast, since the epidermis of the transplant may curl up. Record in your notes the orientation in which the transplant was implanted, or state that the orientation was lost. Check repeatedly whether the glass bridge is in place.

7. After 20–30 minutes, lift the glass bridge gently and remove with the glass needle all loose cells adhering to the edges of the transplant. If healing is not yet completed, replace the glass bridge for another 10–20 minutes. Lift the embryo out of the groove, using the hair loop. Suck it very gently in a wide-mouthed pipette and transfer it to a caster or small paraffined paper cup filled with *dilute* medium. Dip the pipette under the water surface before releasing the embryo. Place the embryo right side up.

8. Clean the donor embryo and transfer it to the same dish, right side up.

9. Give the embryos a serial number (e.g., "bal. 1"), label the dish, and prepare a record. Carefulness in drafting the protocol is as important as carefulness in the operation. Make sketches of donor and host, indicating the position, orientation, etc., of the transplant.

Example of protocol:

Bal. 1: Ambystoma punctatum
March 11   *donor:* stage 28
           host: stage 27
           trpl: right balancer ectoderm and underlying mesoderm

implanted: ventral to somites 7–9 (refer to sketch) in normal orientation; healed
   after 30 minutes
donor saved; wound beginning to heal

March 13 donor: stage H35 OK; left balancer just visible; wound on right side healed
host: stage H36 OK; both host balancers just visible
trpl: healed; first beginning of outgrowth, in typical direction, etc.

Note all changes in the transplant, particularly time and direction of the outgrowth of the transplanted balancer and, later on, its resorption. Compare with the left balancer of the donor or with normal embryos of the same stage as the donor.

Make 3–4 operations; choose different sites of implantation.

Note.—In rare instances the transplant will form a double balancer. Occasionally the tissue which healed over the wound of the donor will also form a balancer. This is indication of a balancer field.

EXPERIMENT 13

Rotate the transplant 90° or 180°.—Observe carefully (and sketch) the direction of outgrowth of the balancer; compare it with the normal balancer. In order to assure the desired orientation of the transplant, it is essential to vital stain its upper right corner before excision. Is the direction of outgrowth determined exclusively by "intrinsic" factors, or is it influenced by the host?

EXPERIMENT 14

Obtain embryos of different stages.—Transplant from a young donor onto a host that is several stages older, and vice versa. Operate with great care in order to keep the donor alive. Observe the first appearance of the transplanted balancer and compare it with that of the left donor (control) balancer. Likewise observe the time of shedding in the transplant, the host, and the donor (control) balancer. Is the life-cycle of the transplant in any way influenced by the host? (See Kollros, 1940.)

BIBLIOGRAPHY

HARRISON, R. G. 1924. The development of the balancer in *Amblystoma,* studied by the method of transplantation and in relation to the connective-tissue problem. Jour. Exper. Zool., **41**:349.

KOLLROS, J. J. 1940. The disappearance of the balancer in *Amblystoma* larvae. Jour. Exper. Zool., **85**:33.

NICHOLAS, J. S. 1924. The development of the balancer in *Amblystoma tigrinum.* Anat. Rec., **28**:317.

c) TRANSPLANTATION OF FORELIMB PRIMORDIA

Study first the normal development of the forelimbs in *Ambystoma* (Harrison, 1918). In stage H28 and earlier, notice the pronephros swelling immediately beneath somites 3–5 and a short distance posterior to the gill swelling. The prospective forelimb area is represented by ectodermal and mesodermal material immediately ventral to the pronephros, including the ventral slope of the pronephric primordium. In stage H36 the limb bud becomes visible as a prominence separate from the pronephros. In stage H37 it is a distinct bud which points in caudal direction. It is at first cone-shaped and then flattens at its distal end. In stage H41 an indentation at its distal outline marks the two digits, 1 and 2, which grow out rapidly in the succeeding stages. Digits 3 and 4 follow successively at the ulnar border. At the same time, the elbow joint becomes visible. Note the posture of the limb. At first its palmar side faces the flank. Then it rotates forward in the shoulder joint, so that the animal supports itself with the forelimbs when it is at rest. The balancers, which performed this function previously, disappear at the time when the digits touch the ground. Limb-bud transplantations were among the earliest embryonic transplantations. The pioneer work was done by Braus (1904) and Harrison (1907) on anurans in connection with certain problems of nerve outgrowth. Later on, Harrison introduced *Ambystoma* embryos as an unusually favorable object for limb transplantation; since then very extensive experimental work has been done by Harrison and his students and by many other investigators, using the limb bud as an object for the analysis of fundamental problems of determination (reviews in Swett, 1937; Nicholas, 1955).

Detwiler (1933) has shown that the prospective limb material is determined as early as in the late yolk-plug stage. For our purpose it is advisable to use older stages, preferably stages H25–H31. Harrison (1918) has demonstrated that the limb-forming potencies reside in the mesoderm and not in the epidermis of the primordium. Removal of ectoderm does not interfere with limb development, whereas extirpation of the entire limb mesoderm, keeping the ectoderm intact in position, usually results in the lack of a limb. Also, heterotopically transplanted limb mesoderm without ectoderm gives rise to a limb. It is therefore essential for the success of the following experiments to include the mesoderm in the graft as completely as possible.

Occasionally the transplant forms *duplicated* limbs. The duplication may affect only the digits, or it may affect the whole limb, or any intermediate degree of duplication may occur. The double limbs are always mirror images of each other. These duplications are of interest in several respects. First, they prove for an organ primordium what constriction experiments (p. 78) have proved for the whole egg in earlier stages: that at the time of transplantation the individual skeletal, muscle, and other elements were not rigidly determined in a mosaic-like fashion. Second, the mirror imaging of all duplications shows that, once a limb bud segregates into two, there must be a reversal of the symmetry relations of one of the partners under the influence of the other partner. The same mirror imaging is frequently found in the viscera, heart, etc., of naturally occurring and artificially produced double monsters and identical twins, where it is known as "situs inversus" (see p. 80). The problem of symmetry and the causes of symmetry inversion in duplicated limbs are discussed by Harrison (1921).

It is of interest to raise the donor embryos of limb transplantations and to find out whether the extirpated primordium can be regulated. If the donor embryo shows no limb defect and the transplant is entirely resorbed, one may suspect that not the limb primordium proper but adjacent tissue has been transplanted by mistake.

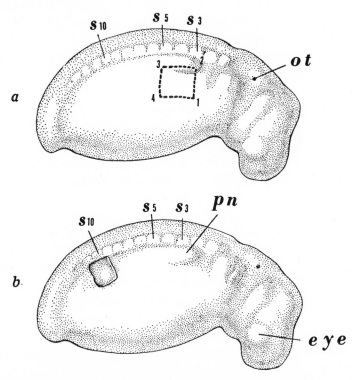

Fig. 22.—Transplantation of a forelimb primordium. a = donor embryo; b = host embryo. 1–2–3–4 = limb area. ot = otocyst; pn = pronephros; $S3$, etc. = somite 3, etc.

EXPERIMENT 15

Material
   Ambystoma (any species), or *Taricha*, or *Diemictylus*, or *Triturus*, stages
      H25–H31
   standard equipment (p. 44)
   0.1 per cent solution of Nile blue sulfate
Procedure (*Fig. 22*)
   1. Prepare at least a dozen embryos of stages H25–H31, preferably stages H28–H30. Select very healthy embryos. Remove all membranes, including the

vitelline membrane, and transfer the embryos in a sterile pipette to sterile dilute medium. Older embryos that begin to show movements must be narcotized in chloretone or MS 222 during the operation (see p. 40).

2. Transfer 2 embryos into the operation dish (full-strength medium) and, with glass rod with ball tip, mold two grooves, side by side, in which the embryos fit when lying right side up. Smooth the edges of the grooves very carefully. Place the embryos in the grooves. Have several glass bridges ready; slip them over the embryo and make sure that they have the proper size and bend.

3. Prepare the host embryo (Fig. 22, b). All transplants should be made to the flank, at some distance posterior to the pronephros swelling of the host, and approximately below somites 8–10. The position of the graft should be in exactly the same level as the host limb, i.e., immediately below the somites. Transplants grafted to a more ventral position, i.e., in the yolk, do not take well and are frequently resorbed or extruded.

Prepare a groove for the transplant. Healing is facilitated if the transplant fits in very tightly. Therefore prepare a relatively small pocket; it is always possible to enlarge it at the moment of implantation. Instead of removing a piece of epidermis, which often results in a wide gap, make merely a slit in ventrodorsal direction, using glass needle and hairloop as described in Experiment 12 under 4 (p. 86). Estimate the length of the slit from the dimensions of the transplant in Figure 22. Remove carefully a considerable amount of mesoderm cells with the tip of the glass needle, so that a rather deep pocket is formed.

4. Extirpate the limb area of the donor (Fig. 22, a). Locate the pronephros swelling. The limb area extends from the third to the fifth somites, immediately ventral to the pronephros swelling, and includes the ventral slope of the latter. With the glass needle make a "stitch" through epidermis and mesoderm along the dorsal border of this area, across the pronephros (line 2–3 in Fig. 22, a), and stroke the hair loop against the needle until a cut is made. Or cut down from the surface. The cut should go deep, and great care should be taken not to loosen the epidermis, which peels off rather easily. Following this, make the other 3 cuts in the same way. Then lift out the entire cut area with the tip of the glass needle, including all mesoderm down to the whitish entoderm. The transplant should be a thick pad of mesoderm, firmly adhering to the epidermis. Avoid losing mesoderm cells during the subsequent transfer. Speed up this part of the operation and the insertion of the transplant in the groove.

Note.—Harrison and his students have made use of iridectomy scissors for extirpations. Operations with this instrument are probably easier, but iridectomy scissors are expensive and therefore usually not available for class use.

5. For implantation, transfer the transplant on the tip of the needle to the

hole in the host; proceed with the greatest care and try not to lose the orientation of the transplant. If necessary drop the transplant near the host without changing its orientation and enlarge the hole. Implant the graft in normal orientation, press it into the hole with the glass needle or the hair loop, and cover it quickly with a glass bridge. Press the bridge firmly against the transplant.

6. Give the embryo a protocol number, make a sketch, and take a careful record, including data on the amount of mesoderm transplanted and the orientation of the graft.

7. After a half-hour remove the glass bridge very cautiously. If the transplant has not healed in properly, place the bridge back for another half-hour. The danger of damaging the embryo by prolonged pressure is less than the chance of losing an improperly healed transplant, which is usually extruded.

8. Transfer the embryo in a wide-mouthed pipette to a paraffined paper cup half-filled with *dilute* medium; clean the wound of the donor embryo of adhering cells and transfer it to the same or to another dish. Label the dish.

Note.—Make 3 or 4 operations of the same kind.

9. During the following weeks observe both host and donor frequently. Narcotize both and study them in the narcotic. Take careful protocols and make sketches of all changes that you observe on the transplant and on the limb region of the donor. Compare the development of the transplant with that of the host limb and with the left forelimb of the donor. Watch carefully for a possible duplication of the transplant; try to detect and sketch it at its inception. This will help in the later interpretation of the symmetry relations.

d) LIMB TRANSPLANTATION WITH INVERSION OF AXES

The origin of polarization and of symmetry relations in an organism or in an organ is one of the major problems in experimental embryology. Harrison (1921) in a classical study analyzed this problem by transplanting limb primordia in such a way that their axes would not coincide with those of the host embryo. In a limb primordium Harrison distinguishes 3 axes, the anterior-posterior (*ap*) axis, the dorsoventral (*dv*) axis, and the mediolateral (*ml*) axis, which coincide with the corresponding axes of the embryo. Left primordia were transplanted to the right flank (Fig. 23, *a* and *c*), or right primordia were rotated 180°, but kept on the same side (Fig. 23, *d*). Transplantations from one side to the other can be done in two ways: either by moving the transplant over the back, so to speak (Fig. 23, *a*), in which case the *dv*-axis is inverted with respect to the host but the *ap*-axes of the host and transplant coincide (*aadv*-orientation, in Harrison's terminology); or by shifting the transplant around the tail, so to speak (Fig. 23, *c*), in which case the *ap*-axis is reversed, but the *dv*-axis is not, (*apdd*-orientation). Rotation by 180°, on the same side,

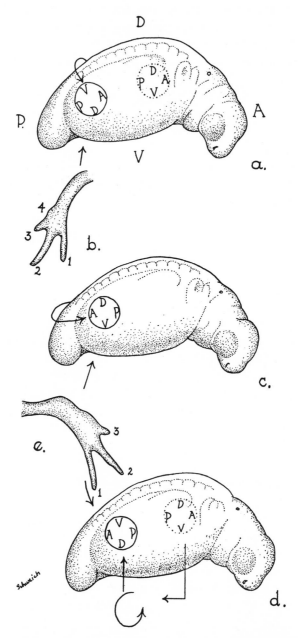

FIG. 23.—Limb transplantations with inversion of axes. $a =$ transplantation of a left forelimb primordium to the right flank, with inversion of the dv-axis ($aadv$-orientation). $A =$ anterior; $P =$ posterior; $D =$ dorsal; $V =$ ventral. The dotted circle and the letters in it indicate the position and axes of the host forelimb; the solid circle and the letters in it indicate the transplant and its axes. $b =$ the transplant resulting from this operation; $c =$ transplantation of a left forelimb primordium to the right flank with inversion of the ap-axis ($apdd$-orientation); $d =$ transplantation of a right forelimb primordium to the right flank, after rotation of 180° ($apdv$-orientation); $e =$ the transplant, resulting from operations c and d (modified, after Swett, 1937).

results in an *apdv*-orientation. Briefly, the results were as follows: The *ap*-axis is irrreversibly fixed. In all instances a transplant in *ap*-orientation grows forward instead of caudad (Fig. 23, *e*). It follows its original trend, uninfluenced by adjacent tissues. The *dv*-axis, however, is not irreversibly fixed, up to stage H32 (in *A. punctatum*). Transplants in *dv*-orientation behave as if they were in a *dd*-orientation, with the first digit growing outward. It can be concluded that the *dv*-axis becomes polarized by influences from adjacent host tissue. This explains the startling phenomenon that, in certain combinations, a left primordium will give rise to a right limb (for instance, in operation, Fig. 23, *a*, *b*), or a right primordium can be made to form a left limb, even if it stays on the right flank (Fig. 23, *d*, *e*). From stage H35 on, the *dv*-axis is also irreversibly fixed. Stages H33 and H34 are transitional stages. For all details see Harrison (1921) and the review of Swett (1937). The experiments clearly illustrate a point which was emphasized on page 84, viz., a primordium may self-differentiate with respect to one characteristic and, at the same time, be dependent on extrinsic factors in other respects.

EXPERIMENT 16: REVERSAL OF THE *dv*-AXIS

Material

Ambystoma, not older than stage H31, preferably younger
standard equipment (p. 44)

Procedure

In order to facilitate the orientation of the transplant, vital-stain the anterior border of the *left* forelimb primordium. Operate as in Experiment 15. Implant to the right flank. Orient the transplant as in Figure 23, *a*. Fit the anterior (marked) border of the transplant to the anterior border of the implantation groove in the host. Note the direction of outgrowth.

EXPERIMENT 17: REVERSAL OF THE *ap*-AXIS

Procedure as before, but fit the anterior (vital-stained) border of the transplant to the posterior border of the implantation groove (Fig. 23, *c*).

EXPERIMENT 18: ROTATION 180°

Proceed as indicated in Figure 23, *d*. What do you expect? How do the results compare with those of the preceding experiments?

BIBLIOGRAPHY (*c–d*)

BRAUS, H. 1904. Einige Ergebnisse der Transplantation von Organanlagen bei Bombinator-Larven. Verh. d. anat. Gessellsch., **18**:53.
DETWILER, S. R. 1933. On the time of determination of the anteroposterior axis of the forelimb in *Amblystoma*. Jour. Exper. Zool., **64**:405.

HARRISON, R. G. 1907. Experiments in transplanting limbs and their bearing upon the problems of the development of nerves. Jour. Exper. Zool., **4**:239.

——. 1918. Experiments on the development of the forelimb of *Amblystoma,* a self-differentiating equipotential system. *Ibid.,* **25**:413.

——. 1921. On relations of symmetry in transplanted limbs. *Ibid.,* **32**:1.

NICHOLAS, J. S. 1955. Limb and girdle. In WILLIER, WEISS, and HAMBURGER (eds.), Analysis of development. Philadelphia: Saunders.

SWETT, F. H. 1937. Determination of limb-axes. Quart. Rev. Biol., **12**:322.

e) TRANSPLANTATION OF GILL PRIMORDIA

The external gills of salamander larvae consist of three branches with secondary filaments. They are fully developed in stage H41. In the stage series (Fig. 45) trace them to earlier stages. In tail-bud stages as early as stage H25 or stage H26 they are clearly distinguishable as lateral swellings on the head, slightly ventral and posterior to the optic vesicle. Familiarize yourself with the normal development of gills.

Harrison (1921) has shown that the gills of *A. maculatum* are determined as early as stage H21. All three germ layers contribute to the formation of the gills. The respective role of each one of them in the determination of the size and shape of gills has been investigated by means of heterotopic, heteroplastic, and xenoplastic[13] transplantation of the three components separately. The considerable literature on this subject is discussed in Severinghaus (1930) and Rotmann (1935). The following experiments will demonstrate that the three-layered gill swelling is self-differentiating in its gross morphology in early tail-bud stages, that is, long before visible differentiation takes place.

EXPERIMENT 19

Material

   Ambystoma, any species, stages H26–H29

   standard equipment (p. 44)

Procedure

1. Select two embryos of approximately the same stage. Remove all membranes. Place them side by side in two grooves in the operating dish (as in Experiment 12, sections 1–3), right side up. Operate in full-strength culture medium.

2. *Prepare the host embryo.*—With glass needle and hair loop prepare a groove in the flank of the host embryo. Choose one of the following sites: posterior or ventral to anterior limb bud; immediately ventral to somites 9–12; in the place of the eye. For this and the following procedure follow the technique described in Experiment 12, under sections 4–8.

---

[13] Heterotopic = transplantation to a different position; heteroplastic = transplantation between embryos belonging to different species; xenoplastic = transplantation between embryos belonging to different genera, families, or more distant taxonomic categories.

3. *Extirpation of the gill primordium.*—Cut out the larger part of the gill swelling, using glass needle and hair loop. Cut very deeply, so that the pharyngeal cavity is exposed. Lift out the block of tissue and transfer it cautiously to the site of implantation, using the tip of the glass needle or the hair loop.

4. Enlarge the hole in the host embryo if necessary. Fit the transplant in and hold it in position with a glass bridge for 30 minutes or longer.

5. After the transplant is healed in, lift the glass bridge cautiously, clean the edges of the wound, and transfer the embryo to a dish filled with dilute culture medium.

6. Take a record; note the orientation of the transplant. Give the embryo a serial number. Operate 3–5 embryos in the same way. In some of them orient the transplant in inverted position.

7. On the following day observe and record all changes in the transplant. Compare its development with that of the host gills. In which orientation do the transplanted gills grow out? Are they of normal size and shape? Are they vascularized? They will be resorbed eventually.

Further suggestions.—Study the papers of Harrison, Severinghaus, and Rotmann and repeat some of the experiments in which ectoderm alone or mesoderm alone was transplanted or rotated.

BIBLIOGRAPHY

HARRISON, R. G. 1921. Experiments on the development of the gills in the amphibian embryo. Biol. Bull., **41**:156.

ROTMANN, E. 1935. Der Anteil von Induktor und reagierendem Gewebe an der Entwicklung der Kiemen und ihrer Gefässe. Arch. f. Entw'mech., **133**:225.

SEVERINGHAUS, A. E. 1930. Gill development in *Amblystoma punctatum*. Jour. Exper. Zool., **56**:1.

4. ISOLATION (EXPLANTATION) EXPERIMENTS

The most rigid test for the inherent differentiation capacities of an embryonic area is its performance in complete isolation from other embryonic parts, in a culture medium that permits adequate differentiation. Such a medium was devised for amphibian material by Holtfreter (1931). The "Holtfreter solution" (and other similar solutions, see p. 34) is a balanced, non-nutritive salt solution, the nutritive material being supplied by the yolk content of the cells. It permits the differentiation of isolated fragments of amphibian embryos of any stage and of any size, ranging from individual cells or small clusters to entire heads or tails.

Using the explantation method, Holtfreter (1938) has made a comprehensive analysis of the differentiation potencies of all parts of the early urodelan and anuran gastrula, when reared in complete isolation, and the analysis has been extended by him and others to later stages. Explantation has been used with particular success for the analysis of embryonic induction, in combination

97

with the "sandwich method" (Holtfreter, 1936). In this experiment, materials to be tested for their inductive capacity, such as the organizer or living or dead adult tissues, or extracts absorbed in agar, are wrapped in a piece of prospective gastrula ectoderm, which by fusion of the free edges forms an ectodermal vesicle. If all precautions are taken, these vesicles survive over long periods and form a variety of structures and organs under the stimulus of the inclosed inductors. In this way, regional differences in the inductivity of the archenteron roof, interactions between tissues belonging to taxonomically different groups, and the chemical properties of inductors have been investigated (review of these results in Holtfreter and Hamburger, 1955). This method has one advantage over intra-embryonic transplantations: all influences of the host embryo are excluded.

Although the "sandwich experiment" is not particularly difficult, it is not very suitable for classroom experiments, largely because the results cannot be evaluated properly without sectioning of the material. However, it is suggested that the experiment be demonstrated by the instructor, using the directions in the original literature. The following data may be of help: A large piece of prospective ectoderm of a young gastrula is placed on an operation dish with agar bottom, outer surface facing downward, and the inductor—as, for instance, upper blastoporal lip—is placed in the middle of the piece and the edges are folded up to envelop the isolate. The edges are gently pressed together to facilitate healing; the vesicle is kept in full-strength medium.

Following again the lead of Holtfreter, great strides have been made in studies of complete dissociation and reaggregation of embryonic cells and in recombinations of different types of dissociated cells (see Townes and Holtfreter, 1955, where the technique is briefly described).

The following exercises have a more limited scope: they are supposed to demonstrate the effectiveness of the isolation method and the capacity of large parts of the neurula and later stages to proceed with their development independently of the rest of the embryo. In using the convenient term "self-differentiation" to designate this capacity, one should be aware of its lack of precision (see p. 84).

a) Medullary Plate

EXPERIMENT 20: ISOLATION OF THE MEDULLARY PLATE WITH
UNDERLYING MESODERM (Fig. 24)

Material

Ambystoma, stages H15–17

Rana, any species, stage 14

standard equipment.—Prepare *special glass needles* that are somewhat
   stronger and slightly longer than the ones used for transplantations

Note.—Use exclusively concentrated medium for rearing of explants.

Procedure

1. Prepare a shallow groove in the operation dish, just deep enough to hold the embryo in position. Make a cut a short distance lateral to the neural folds, all around the embryo, including the blastopore (Fig. 24). Cut rather deeply into the archenteron and not just in the epidermis. If necessary, rub the hair loop against the glass needle to cut through. Before cutting around the caudal end, lift the medullary plate up and observe the germ-layer arrangement. Notice the prospective notochord in the mid-line of the under surface and the endoderm adhering to it rather tightly on both sides. Remove the endoderm mantle along lines rather close to the notochord and also remove the large, loose endoderm cells. Leave the mesoderm intact beneath the medullary plate.

2. Immediately transfer the isolate to an agar dish with concentrated solution. You may rear several explants in one dish. Discard the ventral half if it was seriously injured during the operation; otherwise transfer it to another dish.

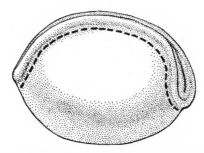

Fig. 24.—Isolation of medullary plate, along the dotted line

3. During the following days observe the differentiation of the axial organs in the dorsal isolates, such as parts of the brain, optic vesicles, somites. Observe the conspicuous elongation and particularly the outgrowth of the tail. The surface of the ventral parts is covered by the "surface coat" (Holtfreter, 1943) that protects the mesoderm and endoderm from dissociation. Ventral parts, raised for a week, may show peristalsis in the non-innervated floor of the gut and heart beat. Make 5–8 isolates of this type.

EXPERIMENT 21: ISOLATION OF THE POSTERIOR ONE-THIRD OF THE MEDULLARY PLATE

Make a deep cut across the medullary plate, separating the anterior two-thirds from the posterior third. Isolate the caudal part, including the blastoporal region, as in the preceding experiment; lift it out and discard the rest of the embryo.

Transfer the explant to a dish with concentrated solution. Make a sketch of the operation. During the following days observe the development of an isolated tail, including tail fins. Read Holtfreter and Hamburger (1955) with reference to tail formation. Remember that the posterior one-fifth of the medullary plate is mesoderm (prospective tail somite material).

99

b) TAIL-BUD STAGE

EXPERIMENT 22: ISOLATION OF HEADS AND TAILS IN TAIL-BUD STAGE

Material

Ambystoma, stages H21–28

strong, rather long glass needles or a steel knife (prepared by sharpening a sewing needle) or a pair of iridectomy scissors (p. 9)

Procedure

1. Place the embryo in a shallow groove. Transect either anterior or posterior to the gill region and at the base of the tail bud. Discard the trunk piece. On a sketch indicate the levels of amputation.

2. Transfer the head and tail pieces to separate dishes. Repeat the operation at the same levels and rear all heads and all tails together, not more than 4 or 5 in the same dish. Discard disintegrating pieces at once.

3. Observe the differentiation of the isolates and compare them with normal controls. Make sketches. Note that the endoderm is covered by cells which have a surface coat. Other endoderm cells not incorporated in the surface-coated layer are discharged. In older tails, contractions may be observed, obviously as a result of local reflexes.

BIBLIOGRAPHY

HOLTFRETER, J. 1931. Über die Aufzucht isolierter Teile des Amphibien-Keimes. II. Arch. f. Entw'mech., **124**:404.

———. 1936. Regionale Inductionen in xenoplastisch zusammengesetzten Explantaten. *Ibid.*, **134**:466.

———. 1938. Differenzierungspotenzen isolierter Teile der Urodelengastrula. *Ibid.*, **138**:522.

———. 1943. Properties and function of the surface coat in amphibian embryos. Jour. Exper. Zool., **93**:251.

——— and V. HAMBURGER. 1955. Amphibians. In WILLIER, WEISS, and HAMBURGER (eds.), Analysis of development. Philadelphia: Saunders.

TOWNES, P. L., and H. HOLTFRETER. 1955. Directed movements and selective adhesion of embryonic amphibian cells. Jour. Exper. Zool., **128**:53.

5. REGULATIVE PROPERTIES OF ORGAN PRIMORDIA (MORPHOGENETIC FIELDS)

a) INTRODUCTORY REMARKS: TERMINOLOGY

In the neurula stage many regions of the amphibian embryo have acquired a considerable degree of self-differentiating capacity. This holds for the limb-forming area; the eye-forming area; the nose, ear, heart, balancer region; etc. These areas have peculiar properties. First of all, they show a high regulative power. When part of a limb, eye, or heart primordium, etc., is transplanted, the transplant will tend to form a whole structure, as will the fragment that was left behind in the donor. In this respect the organ primordia resemble the egg in the 2- or 4-cell stage. They are not composed of a mosaic pattern of smaller, self-differentiating, and specialized units. On the contrary, each part contains within itself a full complement of all factors which are necessary for the formation of a whole. Driesch called such systems "harmonious equipotential systems." If any sufficiently large part of such a system is potentially capable of forming the whole organ, yet only one proportionate limb, eye, or heart develops eventually, then rigid restrictions of potencies must be imposed on the parts. They are assigned to limited, specific tasks within the framework of a whole, and mutual adjustments between the parts must take place. At a time when the limb area as a whole is self-differentiating, as is shown by transplantation experiments (p. 89), the finer structural details within this area, such as individual skeletal elements, muscles, etc., are not yet determined; they gradually become established, in later stages, by mutual interactions of the parts and possibly through other mechanisms. Harmonious equipotential systems illustrate the epigenetic nature of development as well as the relativity of the terms "self-differentiation" and "determination" (see p. 84).

The organ-forming areas which are thus blocked out in the rough have at first no distinct boundaries. The capacity for limb formation in the tail-bud stage, or eye formation in the neurula, may extend beyond the cell area, which, in normal development, will actually form the limb or the eye. This was demonstrated by experiments in which the entire prospective limb- or eye-forming area was extirpated, yet a limb or an eye was formed by adjacent cells, which closed the wound. Finally, within each primordium there seems to exist a gradient of organ-forming capacity with a peak in the center of the field and a gradual decline toward the periphery. Embryonic areas that exhibit the following four characteristics are called "morphogenetic fields": (1) they are self-differentiating systems, as shown by heterotopic transplantation; (2) they are regulative systems, as shown by the formation of normal organs after removal or transplantation of half-primordia or after superimposition of two whole primordia; (3) the specific organ-forming potencies extend beyond the borders of the prospective organ-forming areas; and (4) these self-differentiating regulative areas are gradient fields. For further discussions of the field concept see the books by Spemann, Waddington, and Weiss (p. xvii).

In the following experiments the properties of morphogenetic fields will be illustrated by experiments on the limb, the heart, and the eye primordia.

b) EXTIRPATIONS ON THE LIMB FIELD

The first extensive analysis of field properties was made on the forelimb of *Ambystoma* by Harrison (1918). In tail-bud stages the limb area is a disk immediately ventral to the pronephros, extending from the anterior border of the third somite to the posterior border of the fifth somite. Its dorsal-most part covers the ventral part of the pronephros (Fig. 22, *a*). The limb-forming potencies reside in the mesodermal cells of this area.

Harrison first made a systematic potency test of half-disks: anterior, posterior, dorsal, and ventral halves were extirpated. It was found that any half-disk is capable of forming a whole limb, although the percentage of normal limbs resulting from the operation varied considerably. Detwiler (1918) supplemented these experiments by heterotopic transplantation of dorsal or of ventral half-disks, both of which gave rise to normal limbs. The limb area has thus been shown to be a "self-differentiating harmonious equipotential system," as the title of Harrison's paper indicates. Next, the entire limb disk was removed. Normal limbs developed from cells which migrated into the wound from the periphery. When the diameter of the extirpated disk was increased from 3 to 4 and $4\frac{1}{2}$ somites, normal limbs were still formed in a certain percentage of cases. When the amount of extirpated tissue was further increased, no regulation took place. The percentage of regulating limbs was lower when larger disks were removed or when the wound was thoroughly cleaned of mesoderm cells. Thus it is shown that the limb-forming potencies extend beyond the area which actually enters into limb formation (*i.e.,* the prospective limb area) and that they are higher in the center than at the periphery.

The student should consult the paper of Harrison (1918) for all details.

Material for Experiments 23–26

Ambystoma, any stage between H24 and H30

standard equipment (p. 44)

Experimental procedure for Experiments 23–26

Operate in *full-strength* culture medium. Operate always on the right side of the embryo. Narcotize in chloretone 1:3,000 or MS 222, 1:5,000 if necessary. Proceed as follows:

1. Choose a number of healthy tail-bud stages. Remove all membranes. Wash in sterile culture medium.

2. Transfer one embryo to the operation dish. Prepare a groove of adequate size for the embryo to fit right side up. Locate the pronephros swelling and the limb region (Fig. 22, *a*).

3. With the glass needle (or the iridectomy scissors) cut out the desired part of the limb area; make a rectangular hole if you use the glass needle. Allow wound-healing in concentrated medium for 15–30 minutes.

4. Make a careful sketch, prepare a protocol, label the embryo, and transfer it to a dish containing *dilute* solution.

5. Observe the healing of the wound in the following hours and the differentiation of the limb in the following weeks. Make sketches and take careful protocols. Does the regulating limb catch up with the left (control) limb?

EXPERIMENT 23

Removal of the dorsal half of the limb area.—Cut out the dorsal half of the square *1–2–3–4* in Figure 22, *a*. Make 3–5 operations. In some cases clean the wound carefully of all mesoderm cells with the tip of the glass needle; in other cases leave some mesoderm behind. Record in each instance the amount of mesoderm left in the wound. Note differences in the regulation.

EXPERIMENT 24

Removal of the anterior half of the square *1–2–3–4* in Figure 22, *a*.

EXPERIMENT 25

Removal of the entire prospective limb area, 3 somites in diameter (*1–2–3–4* in Fig. 22, *a*).

EXPERIMENT 26

Removal of an area 4 somites in diameter, centering ventrally to the fourth somite.

Note.—In evaluating the results, one must bear in mind that not all quadrants of the limb disk share equally in the formation of the limb itself. For instance, the ventral half contributes less than the dorsal half. The prospective significance of the different sectors has been worked out by Swett (1923), using the vital-staining method.

BIBLIOGRAPHY

Detwiler, S. R. 1918. Experiments on the development of the shoulder girdle and the anterior limb of *Amblystoma punctatum*. Jour. Exper. Zool., **25**:499.
Harrison, R. G. 1918. Experiments on the development of the forelimb of *Amblystoma*, a self-differentiating equipotential system. Jour. Exper. Zool., **25**:413.
Swett, F. H. 1923. The prospective significance of the cells contained in the four quadrants of the primitive limb disc in *Amblystoma*. Jour. Exper. Zool., **37**:207.

c) FORMATION OF TWO HEARTS

The heart is formed by two originally separate lateral primordia, the free ventral edges of the left and right hypomere. In *Amblystoma*, stage H27, the latter have approached the mid-line and given off a small number of cells, situated in the mid-line. These cells, the primordia of the endocardium, signal the beginning of visible heart formation. The outline of the right heart-forming area at this stage is indicated in Figure 25, *c*. In stage H33, the endocardial tube is formed but not yet curved. The formation of the different subdivisions of the heart by differential growth occurs in the subsequent stages. Circulation begins at about stages H36–H37; the first spontaneous pulsations begin in stage H34. The student should review details of heart development in textbooks of embryology and consult Copenhaver (1926, 1939, 1955) before starting the experimental work. For the experimenter, it is important to be acquainted with the localization of the heart primordia in early stages and to realize the extensive movements which the prospective heart-forming material undergoes. It can be traced to the inner marginal zone of the gastrula, that is, the deeper layer of the lateral lip of the crescent-shaped blastopore. In the late neurula the primordia are in a dorsolateral position, and in stage 22 they are still a considerable distance apart from each other (see Copenhaver, 1955, Fig. 157, p. 441).

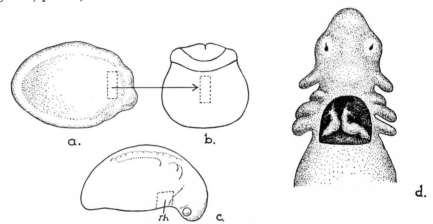

FIG. 25.—Production of two hearts out of one primordium (*c, d,* after Copenhaver, 1926). *a =* donor embryo; the dotted lines indicate the strip of tissue (gill area) which is implanted in the region indicated in *b* by dotted lines. *b =* host embryo; *d =* heart region of host embryo, dissected (note that the two hearts are mirror images of each other); *c =* right half of the prospective heart area (*rh*) is stage 27.

The heart-forming material and the surrounding tissue have all the properties of a morphogenetic field up to relatively advanced tail-bud stages. This was demonstrated by the same potency tests that were applied to the limb primordium (p. 101).

1. *Relative self-differentiation.*—Following the early pioneer work of Ekman and Stoehr, the explantation experiments of Bacon (1945) and the heterotopic transplantations of Copenhaver (1926) have demonstrated considerable self-differentiation capacities of the heart-forming material. Explants of heart mesoderm, from neurula stages on, can form tubes which are subdivided into 2 or 3 parts and show S-shaped curvature and pulsation. Heterotopic transplantation of the heart primordium at stage H28 results in the formation of a fairly well differentiated, pulsating heart. However, such hearts are never completely normal, although they may be incorporated in the blood stream of the host, and there is no doubt but that the mechanical conditions of the environment (pericardial cavity, liver, etc.) and the blood pressure have an influence

104

on the form of the curvature and the later phases of differentiation of the heart. This point illustrates again the relativity of the concept of "self-differentiation."

2. *Regulative properties.*—The peculiarity of heart formation from two originally widely separate primordia makes this material ideally suited for the demonstration of regulation: If the union of the two lateral primordia is prevented by implantation of foreign tissue mid-ventrally between them, then each of the two can form a whole heart (Ekman, 1925; Copenhaver, 1926). Such double hearts usually pulsate with different rates. They are often mirror images of each other, the left heart showing the typical asymmetry and the right heart showing an inversion of symmetry (*situs inversus cordis,* see Fig. 25, *d* herein and discussion in Copenhaver, 1955). The regulative capacity can also be demonstrated by extirpation of parts of primordia. Anterior, posterior, left, and right halves can form more or less typical whole structures. Such hearts from fragments of heart material approach normal tubes with typical subdivisions. This experiment can be done successfully up to relatively late stages (H33) when the heart tube is already formed (Copenhaver, 1926).

3. *The heart field extends beyond the limits of the prospective heart-forming area.*—The complete extirpation of the material that normally forms the heart, in stage H27 of *Ambystoma,* is usually followed by the formation of one or two hearts. One can extirpate an even larger area of lateral plate mesoderm and still obtain small single or double hearts (Copenhaver, 1926, 1955, Fig. 158, p. 442).

The following experiments illustrate points 2 and 3.

EXPERIMENT 27: BLOCKING OF THE FUSION OF LEFT AND RIGHT PRIMORDIA

Material

Ambystoma or *Rana* embryos (For hosts use medullary-plate or medullary-fold stages; for donors use late neurulae or early tail-bud stages.)

standard equipment (p. 44)

Procedure

1. Take donor and host out of all membranes and place them side by side in grooves in an operating dish. Orient the donor right side up and the host ventral side up. Operate in concentrated medium.

2. With the glass needle make a longitudinal slit in the median ventral line of the head of the host. The slit should extend from the outer edge of the medullary fold backward to about one-third of the entire length of the embryo. Cut deeply and make a wide gap without injuring the heart mesoderm to the left and the right (Fig. 25, *b*).

3. The tissue that is to serve as a block must be self-differentiating, or else it might be incorporated in the host heart. Therefore slightly older donors are

preferable. The prospective gill region was found to be suitable as a block; but any other tissue—for instance, somites—will serve the same purpose. With a glass needle cut out a long and narrow strip from the prospective gill area of the donor (Fig. 25, *a*). The strip should include all three germ layers. Cut deeply until the pharyngeal cavity is reached. Implant this strip in the slit of the host in a longitudinal direction. Take care that the epidermis of the transplant is in close contact with that of the host. Place a glass bridge over the transplant for 30 minutes or longer.[14]

4. Remove the glass bridge after the transplant has healed in; discard the donor; place the host in another dish in dilute medium. Rear them together with a few unoperated embryos of host age. Take a careful record.

Note.—Make 3 or more operations.

5. Terminate the experiment after 3–4 days, when heart pulsations are clearly noticeable in control embryos. Carefully scrutinize the operated animals for heart pulsations, which may be very faint. For this purpose, narcotize the embryos; place them in grooves in an operation dish, ventral side up. The epidermis covering the heart region becomes gradually transparent. If it is not yet transparent, then it should be dissected. Practice the in vivo dissection first on one or two unoperated embryos. Use a strong glass needle, iridectomy scissors, or watchmaker forceps with very sharp points. Carefully avoid damage to the beating hearts; expose them completely. The double hearts may be in a far dorsal position, higher up than in Fig. 25, *d*, and they may be very small. Do they beat synchronously? Take careful notes.

6. In order to study the structure of the hearts, it is advisable to expose them by removing all adhering mesenchyme cells. This can be done best after fixation. When all observations on the living specimens are completed, fix the dissected embryos and the controls in 10 per cent formaldehyde + 5 per cent aqueous solution of nitric acid. Dissect carefully with the tip of the glass needle or watchmaker forceps until the heart is completely cleaned and exposed. Study the different parts and the curvature of the double hearts and compare them with controls. Study their symmetry relations. Make sketches and take notes. If the block did not extend sufficiently far anterior or posterior, the heart may be only partially duplicated.

d) PARTIAL AND TOTAL REMOVAL OF THE PROSPECTIVE HEART REGION

EXPERIMENT 28

Material

Ambystoma, stages H26–H28

standard equipment (p. 44)

---

[14] It is possible to obtain double hearts without implantation of a tissue block, by preventing the deep median incision from healing together, thus creating an open fistula.

Procedure

1. Remove all membranes. Place the embryo in a groove in the operation dish, ventral side up.

2. With a glass needle remove the right half of the heart area as indicated in Figure 25, *c*. Apply the technique described in Experiment 12 under section 5 (pp. 87). Extirpate ectoderm and mesoderm. Do not cover the wound. Make several operations.

3. Transfer the embryos to paraffined paper cups (dilute medium) and allow them to develop for several days. Notice the heart beat.

4. Fix and dissect the embryos from the ventral side with a strong glass needle, as in Experiment 27, section 6. Take protocols, make sketches.

EXPERIMENT 29: REMOVAL OF THE ENTIRE PROSPECTIVE HEART REGION

Procedure

Proceed as in Experiment 28. Remove area *rh* (Fig. 25, *c*) and the corresponding area on the left side.

BIBLIOGRAPHY (*c–d*)

BACON, R. 1945. Selfdifferentiation and induction in the heart of *Amblystoma*. Jour. Exper. Zool., **98**:87.

COPENHAVER, W. M. 1926. Experiments on the development of the heart of *Amblystoma punctatum*. Jour. Exper. Zool., **43**:321.

———. 1939. Initiation of beat and intrinsic contraction rates in the different parts of the *Amblystoma* heart. *Ibid.*, **80**:193.

———. 1955. Heart, etc. In WILLIER, WEISS, and HAMBURGER (eds.), Analysis of development. Philadelphia: Saunders.

EKMAN, G. 1925. Experimentelle Beiträge zur Herzentwicklung der Amphibien. Arch. f. Entw'mech., **106**:320.

———. 1929. Experimentelle Untersuchungen über die früheste Herzentwicklung bei *Rana fusca. Ibid.*, **116**:327.

STOEHR, P. 1925. Entstehung der Herzform. Arch. f. Entw'mech., **106**:409.

e) EXTIRPATION OF PARTS OF THE EYE-FORMING REGION
IN THE NEURULA

The prospective eye-forming area in the neurula has been localized by Manchot (1929) and Woerdeman (1929), using the method of vital staining (see p. 64 and Fig. 26). In the medullary-plate stage, the prospective eye regions are located near the median line. In the medullary-fold stage, they have moved apart and border on the inner edge of the folds. The narrow median strip between the two eye regions represents the chiasma region. While the two eye-forming regions move apart, material which was located more posteriorly moves forward and forms that part of the brain floor which eventually separates the eyes.

The anterior part of the medullary plate represents a "forebrain-eye field" in the sense defined above. It shows relative self-differentiation into eye and forebrain when transplanted and, at the same time, has regulative properties. The two eye-forming regions are not yet rigidly determined; in fact, eye-forming potentialities extend beyond the prospective eye-forming areas. There seems to be a mediolateral gradient of eye-forming capacities. These conclusions are based primarily on the extensive transplantation experiments of H. B. Adelmann (1929*a*, 1929*b*, 1930) and O. Mangold (see 1931). The student is referred to the review by Adelmann (1936) concerning *Ambystoma*. To summarize the results of Adelmann:

If a median strip of the anterior medullary plate about $\frac{1}{3}$–$\frac{1}{4}$ of the greatest width of the neural plate (Fig. 26) is transplanted to the flank of another embryo, the wound in the donor will heal and two eyes may be formed by regula-

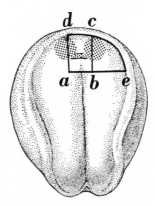

Fig. 26.—Extirpations in the eye field of the medullary-fold stage. The dotted areas indicate the prospective eye-forming regions (see text).

tion of the lateral parts that contain only part of the prospective eye-forming material. The transplant may also form 1 or 2 eyes, in addition to some forebrain material. Thus the forebrain-eye field is capable of forming more than 2 eyes. The removal of a lateral $\frac{1}{3}$ may likewise result in a complete regulation. The experiments demonstrate that the pattern of structures in the field is not yet irreversibly fixed. In order to suppress the formation of one eye completely, it is necessary to make a defect which extends to the median line and caudal to the level of the widest portion of the plate. This shows that the eye-forming potencies extend beyond the prospective eye-forming area. A mediolateral gradient of eye-forming potencies was established by comparing the percentages of eye formation from lateral and from median strips. It was as high as 70 per cent for median strips and only 11 per cent for lateral strips under otherwise identical conditions. If the "peak" of eye-forming capacity is in the center of the medullary plate, why are 2 lateral eyes formed in normal development instead of 1 single median eye? Adelmann (1930) has shown that the underlying endomesoderm is responsible for this effect. It creates bilaterality by "reinforcing" the eye potencies in lateral regions. When median strips of the medullary plate were transplanted with and without the endomesodermal substrate (prechordal mesoderm), those with substrate formed 2 eyes in almost 50 per cent of the cases, while those without substrate never formed 2 whole eyes and at best only a single eye. The explanation of the origin of one-eyed monsters (cyclopia) is along these lines (see also Mangold and von Woellwarth, 1950). The presence or absence of the mesodermal substrate should be given special consideration in the following experiments.

Material for experiments 30–33

Any species of *Urodela*, stages corresponding to H14–H16, preferably H15. The following directions are based on *A. punctatum (Note.*—The localization of the eye-forming regions as indicated in Figure 26 holds only for stage 15. In stage 14 these regions are closer to the mid-line and in stage 16 they have shifted more laterally.

standard equipment (p. 44)

EXPERIMENT 30: REMOVAL OF THE MEDIAN ONE-THIRD OF THE ANTERIOR MEDULLARY PLATE WITHOUT SUBSTRATE

Procedure

1. Remove all membranes from a number of healthy neurulae.

2. Prepare a sterile dish with agar bottom; make a shallow groove in the agar and place an embryo in it. Use full-strength culture medium.

3. With a glass needle and hair loop cut out the area *a–b–c–d* in Fig. 26 (about $\frac{1}{3}$–$\frac{1}{4}$ of the width of the medullary plate). Follow the technique described in Experiment 12, section 5 (p. 87). Make the anterior cut very close to the inner edge of the transverse neural fold. Do not cut deeply; with some experience it is not difficult to peel off the medullary plate with the tip of the needle and hair loop without injury to the roof of the archenteron.

4. In a sketch, outline the extirpated area as precisely as possible; note also any injury to the archenteron.

5. Allow the wound to heal in concentrated medium (this may take an hour or longer) and transfer to another sterile agar dish, with dilute medium.

6. Make several identical operations. Keep 3 or 4 unoperated embryos as controls.

7. Observe the development of the eyes during the subsequent days. Compare with those of the controls. Dorsal views will show whether the eyes are of normal size.

8. When the eyes have become pigmented and the cornea transparent, approximately at stage H37 in *Ambystoma,* terminate the experiment. Narcotize the larvae deeply, make a sketch and fix in formaldehyde. Dissect the skin

109

over brain and eyes with a sturdy glass needle or fine forceps (use special instruments for fixed material). Do the same for a control larva. Compare, describe, and sketch any deviations from normal. Note variations in the degree of regulation in different specimens. How could such differences originate? Of particular interest in this experiment and in Experiments 31 and 32 are cases in which small but otherwise typical eyes are formed. They demonstrate a characteristic feature of morphogenetic fields: if material is removed from a field, the remaining part reorganizes itself to form a smaller but complete whole. Compare your results with those of others.

Experiment 31: Removal of a Mediolateral Strip of the Medullary Plate without Substrate

Note.—Whereas Experiment 30 follows the design of Adelmann and others, the following slight modification has one advantage: incomplete regulation of the eye can be easily detected by its smaller size. However, the unoperated side, by supplying material to cover the wound, may in some instances be slightly reduced in size and therefore not be a valid control. It is therefore safer to check with an unoperated control larva.

Procedure.—Remove an area of the same size as in the preceding experiment but start in the mid-line. Follow instructions for Experiment 30.

Experiment 32: Removal of the Lateral One-third of the Medullary Plate without Substrate

Procedure.—Remove area *b–c–e*. Cut along the inner edge of the neural fold from *c* to *e*. Otherwise follow instructions for Experiment 30.

Experiment 33: Removal of the Median One-third of the Medullary Plate with Substrate

Procedure.—Remove area *a–b–c–d* in Fig. 26. Cut deeply down to the archenteron roof and remove the prechordal substrate underneath the medullary plate along with the latter. In all other respects follow instructions for Experiment 30.

Note.—This defect should not result in a complete regulation, but the degree of the deficiency will depend on the size of the extirpated area. Compare the results with those obtained in Experiment 30.

BIBLIOGRAPHY

Adelmann, H. B. 1929*a*. Experimental studies on the development of the eye. I. The effect of the removal of median and lateral areas of the anterior end of the urodelan neural plate on the development of the eyes (*Triton taeniatus* and *Amblystoma punctatum*). Jour. Exper. Zool., **54**:249.

———. 1929*b*. Experimental studies on the development of the eye. II. The eye-forming potencies of the median portions of the urodelan neural plate (*Triton taeniatus* and *Amblystoma punctatum*). *Ibid.*, **54**:291.

———. 1930. Experimental studies on the development of the eye. III. The effect of the substrate (*Unterlagerung*) on the heterotopic development of median and lateral strips of the anterior end of the neural plate of *Amblystoma*. *Ibid.*, **57**:223.

———. 1936. The problem of Cyclopia. Quart. Rev. Biol., **11**:161, 284.

———. 1937. Experimental studies on the development of the eye. IV. The effect of the partial and complete excision of the prechordal substrate on the development of the eyes of *Amblystoma punctatum*. Jour. Exper. Zool., **75**:199.

MANCHOT, E. 1929. Abgrenzung des Augenmaterials und anderer Teilbezirke in der Medullarplatte. Arch. f. Entw'mech., **116**:689.

MANGOLD, O. 1931. Das Determinationsproblem. III. Das Wirbeltier-Auge. Ergebn. d. Biol., **7**:193.

——— and WOELLWARTH, C. VON. 1950. Das Gehirn von Triton. Naturw., **37**:365, 390.

WOERDEMAN, M. W. 1929. Experimentelle Untersuchungen über Lage und Bau der augenbildenden Bezirke in der Medullarplatte beim Axolotl. Arch. f. Entw'mech., **116**:220.

f) PARTIAL AND TOTAL EXTIRPATION OF THE OPTIC VESICLE

In the early tail-bud stages the optic primordium has proceeded to form the optic vesicle. The prospective significance of the different parts of the vesicle, namely, retina, pigment epithelium, stalk, has been mapped by Petersen (1923; see Fig. 27, *b*).

The optic vesicle is still capable of regulation, both in urodeles and in anurans. Even small fragments of the vesicle may form normal, though smaller, eyes (reviews in Mangold, 1931; Twitty, 1955). The prospective retina may replace the prospective pigment epithelium if the latter is removed, and vice versa. The optic vesicle still has field properties. These findings illustrate clearly a point of theoretical importance mentioned above: The optic primordium is self-differentiating as a whole, but its parts (retina, etc.) are not yet self-differentiating units, even in relatively late stages. Determination is a process that continues over a considerable period, during which first the general and then the detailed characters of an organ primordium become irreversibly fixed. The optic vesicle differs from other morphogenetic fields in one respect—eye-forming properties do not transcend the boundaries of the prospective eye area. No eye regeneration occurs when the optic vesicle is entirely extirpated. This result illustrates another general principle to be emphasized further in the chapter on "Regeneration," that regulation and regeneration are properties of fields and not of the organism as a whole. A fragment of a morphogenetic field is capable of restoring the lost parts, but the organism is not capable of restoring a field once it is lost entirely.

EXPERIMENT 34: REMOVAL OF THE DISTAL REGION OF THE OPTIC VESICLE

Material

Rana sylvatica, palustris, stages PM16–PM17 (*R. pipiens* embryos are sticky in these stages and therefore less desirable. They may be used if no other material is available); *Ambystoma,* any species; *Taricha* standard equipment (p. 44)

Procedure

The student is advised to dissect the eyes of normal embryos (fresh or fixed in 10 per cent formaldehyde) before the operations are started.

1. Select a number of healthy embryos; remove all membranes. Place one embryo in a groove in the operation dish, right side up. Operate in full-strength culture medium.

2. Locate the right optic vesicle; it forms a slight bulge on the surface. With the glass needle and hair loop cut out a square piece of epidermis over the eye (*l.e.* in Fig. 27, *a*). Remove the skin. The window should be so large that the optic vesicle (*o.v.*) is clearly exposed.

3. Remove the outer (distal) half of the optic vesicle with the glass needle (cut *a–b* in Fig. 27, *b*). Make sure under the high power that the cavity of

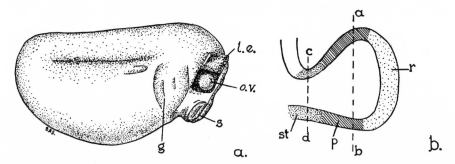

FIG. 27.—Eye extirpations in the tail-bud stage. *a* = the optic vesicle exposed; *g* = gill region; *l.e.* = lens epithelium; *o.v.* = optic vesicle; *s* = suckers; *b* = the prospective areas of the optic vesicle (from Mangold, 1931, after Petersen); *p* = pigment epithelium; *r* = retina; *st* = optic stalk.

the vesicle is exposed. Leave the embryo in full-strength medium until wound-healing is well under way. It is not necessary to cover the wound with foreign epidermis. Adjacent epidermis will grow over.

4. Transfer the embryo to a dish with dilute medium. Take a record.

5. When the cornea over the eyes has become transparent (after 1 week or longer), fix the embryo in 10 per cent formaldehyde and dissect the skin over the eye. Note the degree of regulation, the size, etc., of the operated eye in comparison with the left (control) eye. Make sketches. Make several operations.

EXPERIMENT 35: TOTAL EXTIRPATION OF THE OPTIC VESICLE

Material and procedure as in Experiment 34, except that the entire vesicle is removed by a cut near the brain (*c–d* in Fig. 27, *b*). Make certain under the high power that only the narrow opening of the stalk into the brain, rather than the wide lumen of the optic vesicle, remains. Fix and dissect the embryo after 1 week. Notice the complete absence of the eye.

BIBLIOGRAPHY

Mangold, O. 1931. Das Determinationsproblem. III. Das Wirbeltierauge. Ergebn. d. Biol., 7:193.

Petersen, H. 1923. Berichte über Entwicklungsmechanik I. Ergebn. d. Anat. u. Entw'gesch., 24:327.

Twitty, V. 1955. Eye. In Willier, Weiss, and Hamburger (eds.), Analysis of development. Philadelphia: Saunders.

6. EMBRYONIC INDUCTION

a) INTRODUCTORY REMARKS: TERMINOLOGY

The experiments to be discussed next center around the following problems: Which factors are instrumental in the process of determination? How is the determination of the medullary plate, of the eye, of the balancer, accomplished? There is no one answer to these questions. Different agents are at work in each instance, and each primordium requires a special analysis.

Of the few general mechanisms so far discovered, that of "embryonic induction" is of considerable importance. It may be defined as a process in which one embryonic area, the *inductor,* calls forth a specific differentiation in an adjacent embryonic tissue by contact. The two best analyzed and most widely known cases are the lens induction by the optic vesicle and the induction of the medullary plate by the underlying mesoderm.

The term "induction" includes quite heterogeneous types of interactions, ranging from mere "trigger" actions to highly specific interactions. Induction undoubtedly does not comprise a physiologically uniform group of phenomena. If one bears this in mind, then the use of this convenient term as defined above will do no harm.

Embryonic induction can be demonstrated in two ways: by extirpation and by transplantation. If a causal relationship between two developing structures is suspected, then the removal of one should result in the failure of the other to differentiate However, negative results are not always conclusive, because the failure to differentiate may be due to an unintentional injury of the reacting tissue or to other, non-specific side-effects of the operation. Conclusive evidence for induction can be obtained from transplantation experiments in which the inductor can demonstrate its inductive capacity in a positive way. The transplantation experiments consist essentially in a combination of the structure whose inductive capacity is to be tested with relatively indifferent, that is, not self-differentiating, embryonic tissue. If the latter forms a structure that it would not have formed in the absence of the former, then induction is demonstrated. For instance, in some species the combination of an optic vesicle with flank ectoderm results in lens formation by induction; likewise, the archenteron roof of a late gastrula, when brought in contact with ventral ectoderm of a young gastrula elicits in the latter the

113

formation of a neural tube. Negative results may be caused by the incapacity of the exposed tissue to react. The responsiveness, or *competence,* of an embryonic tissue to react to an inductive stimulus depends on its age, on species characteristics, and on other factors. Hence, the choice of an appropriate test tissue is of importance. The student is referred to discussions of embryonic induction by Spemann (1938), Holtfreter and Hamburger (1955), Waddington (1956), and other texts.

b) FAILURE OF LENS FORMATION AFTER EXTIRPATION OF THE EYE
PRIMORDIUM IN THE MEDULLARY PLATE

The optic cup and the lens originate from two different sources: the former as an evagination of the forebrain, the latter as an invagination of the head epidermis. In the neural-fold stage, the two prospective areas are located at some distance from each other (Fig. 18, *a*). The fact that the lens is formed at the point at which the optic vesicle establishes contact with the overlying epidermis is suggestive of a causal relation between the two. Spemann was the first to test this assumption experimentally. He extirpated the eye primordium in the medullary-plate or optic-vesicle stage and found that no lens would differentiate, although the prospective lens area was left undisturbed. He concluded that lens differentiation is induced by the optic vesicle. His first experiments were made on the European grass frog, *Rana temporaria (fusca).* When another species, *R. esculenta,* was used, a lens, though small and not fully differentiated, was formed in the absence of the optic vesicle, indicating species differences. The lens has since become one of the classical objects for the analysis of embryonic induction. The results of Spemann were confirmed and extended. The major role of the optic primordium in lens induction has been recognized, but the species differences in the behavior of the lens epithelium in the absence of the optic primordium indicate that other factors are involved (reviews in all textbooks; see also reviews by Mangold, 1931; Spemann, 1938; Twitty, 1955; and Ten Cate, 1956).

More recent experiments have contributed to the elucidation of the complex situation. First of all, the notion that the optic vesicle is "the" lens inductor requires revision. Several other tissues adjacent to the lens epithelium during the critical period of lens determination have been implicated as reinforcing auxiliary factors; among them, in the first place, the subjacent head mesoderm and, also, the anterior archenteron roof. We are not dealing with a single inductor but with an *inductor system,* that is, a combination of agents which operate in succession and supplement each other. This concept is probably valid in most, if not all, inductive processes. Furthermore, it was found that the temperature at which the embryos are reared, prior to the operation, is an important factor; in several species, low temperatures greatly enhance formation of lenses in the absence of the optic primordium, though these lenses are never completely normal in size and differentiation. It is conceivable that the cold treatment retards morphological lens development but not its intrinsic biochemical differentiation, or that the action of head mesoderm over a prolonged period subsitutes, in part, for that of the optic vesicle (see Twitty, 1955).

The extirpation of the eye primordium can be done either in the medullary-plate stage or in an early optic-vesicle stage, before a contact between optic vesicle and epidermis is established. Experimentation in the earlier stage has the advantage that the lens-forming area need not be disturbed at all, where-as, in the tail-bud stage, the lens epidermis must be lifted up to get access to the eye and then healed back again.

EXPERIMENT 36

Note.—At room temperature, most American urodeles and anurans form no lenses, or only slight epidermal thickenings, in the absence of the optic primordium. *Taricha torosa* forms small, solid epidermal outgrowths (len-toids) and small vesicles, in a low percentage of cases, at 25° C. (Jacobson, 1958). For a study of induction, cases of abortive lens formation are, of course, as interesting as cases of complete absence of this differentiation. However, epidermal thickenings and lentoids can be observed only on serial sections. To obtain uniform results, it is advisable to rear the embryos in room temperature prior to operation.

Material

> *Rana sylvatica* (stage PM14) or *R. pipiens* (stage Sh14) or corresponding stages of *R. palustris* or *catesbeiana, Ambystoma,* stage H15 or stage H16, or corresponding stages of *Taricha*

Procedure

The aim of this experiment is to remove the eye primordium (part of anterior medullary plate) without disturbing the lens-forming area, which is located just outside the medullary plate or fold (see Fig. 18, *L*). The experiment is identical with Experiment 30 (p. 109) except that a median cut should be made instead of *a–d* and the transverse cut be made slightly posterior to *a–b* (Fig. 26), in order to prevent eye regeneration. Again, first make the median cut, then the cut in direction *b–c*, and finally the cut in direction *c–d*. Carefully avoid any damage to the mesodermal substrate and to the prospective lens area. Follow the technique described for Experiment 30 (p. 109). Operate in full-strength culture medium and allow wound-healing in this solution. Take protocols of the operation. Operate on several embryos.

Fix the larvae in 10 per cent formaldehyde when the swimming stage is reached and the cornea over the left eye is clear. Note the opaque left lens and

115

the absence of a transparent cornea on the right side. Carefully dissect the skin of the right side of the head. Find out if the right eye is completely absent. The presence of a small eye may be the result of an incomplete extirpation and a regulation of the fragment. Note whether a small, whitish, opaque lens is attached to such a regenerated eye. The complete absence of all rudiments of a lens can be definitely established only by sectioning.

c) FAILURE OF LENS FORMATION AFTER EXTIRPATION OF THE OPTIC VESICLE IN EARLY TAIL-BUD STAGES

EXPERIMENT 37

Material

Rana sylvatica, stage PM16, or corresponding stage of R. paluṣtris, or Ambystoma stage H21–23. If only R. pipiens is available, then stage Sh15, or slightly younger, should be used, because in later stages the epidermis adheres tightly to the optic vesicle and the two are difficult to separate.

standard equipment (p. 44).

Procedure

Before starting the operation, locate the optic vesicle on a normal embryo and expose it by removing the epidermis in order to obtain a clear picture of the topographic relationships.

1. Remove all membranes. Place an embryo in a groove in an agar dish together with a well-fitting glass bridge.

2. With the glass needle cut out a square flap of epidermis overlying the optic vesicle, on three sides only, as in Fig. 27, *a*. Reflect the flap and extirpate the optic vesicle at its base. It is essential to avoid injury or curling of the prospective lens epithelium. Turn the flap back; very cautiously flatten it out with hair loop or glass needle, so that the edges come in contact with the adjacent epidermis, and place a glass bridge over it. Control the healing during the following 20–30 minutes.

3. Record the details of the operation and transfer the embryo to a dish with dilute medium. Operate several embryos in the same way.

4. Fix the swimming larvae several days later in 10 per cent formaldehyde. Carefully dissect the skin over both eyes and notice the absence of the right lens in the absence of the right optic cup. Notice the left lens. The lens becomes opaque through fixation and can thus be easily recognized.

d) LENS INDUCTION AFTER REMOVAL OF THE PROSPECTIVE LENS EPITHELIUM

Once a causal relation is established between optic vesicle and lens formation, a number of questions arise concerning the nature of lens induction. For instance, is epidermis from other parts of the embryo "competent" to respond

116

to the stimulus by the optic vesicle? Again, species differences in lens competence were observed: In *R. esculenta* it is limited to the prospective lens area, in *R. pipiens* it is limited to head epidermis, whereas in *R. sylvatica, palustris, catesbeiana* and *Ambystoma punctatum* the trunk epidermis was also found to have "lens competence." The following experiment can therefore be expected to give positive results in all American species. However, if *R. pipiens* is used, stages younger than 15 should be employed, since, from this stage on, the epidermis adheres tightly to the optic vesicle, and it was found that even very small remnants of the lens epithelium that are left behind can regenerate and form a lens, thus vitiating the validity of the experiment (Liedke, 1942).

EXPERIMENT 38

Material

    R. pipiens, stage Sh14, *Rana sylvatica*, PM15–16, corresponding stages of other species of *Rana, Ambystoma* H20–22.

Procedure

1. Remove all membranes.

2. Operate in concentrated medium. Place the embryo in a groove in an agar dish, right side up. With the glass needle, remove a square piece of epidermis that will cover the optic vesicle (*l.e.* in Fig. 27, *a*). Carefully avoid injury to the optic vesicle. Leave the embryo in the concentrated solution for 20–40 minutes. Observe the covering of the wound by adjacent head epidermis.

3. Take a record and transfer the embryo to a paper cup containing dilute solution.

4. After the embryo has reached the swimming stage, fix it in 10 per cent formaldehyde. After a few minutes the lenses will become visible as opaque white structures. Note that the epidermis that has grown over the right eye has become transparent and forms a normal cornea. Dissect the cornea away from both eyes and study the size and shape of the right lens, which has been induced from head epidermis.

BIBLIOGRAPHY

JACOBSON, A. G. 1958. The roles of neural and non-neural tissues in lens induction. Jour. Exper. Zool., **139**:525.

LIEDKE, K. 1942. Lens competence in *Rana pipiens*. Jour. Exper. Zool., **90**:331.

MANGOLD, O. 1931. Das Determinationsproblem. III. Das Wirbeltier-Auge. Ergebn. d. Biol., **7**:193.

SPEMANN, H. 1938. Embryonic development and induction. New Haven: Yale University Press.

TEN CATE, C. 1956. The intrinsic embryonic development. Verh. Koningl. Nederl. Akad. Wetensch., **51**:1.

TWITTY, V. C. 1955. Eye. In WILLIER, WEISS, and HAMBURGER (eds.), Analysis of development. Philadelphia: Saunders.

e) THE ORGANIZER EXPERIMENT: TRANSPLANTATION OF THE
UPPER LIP OF THE BLASTOPORE

Note.—Before starting this experiment read the chapter on the organizer in a textbook. See also the review by Holtfreter and Hamburger (1955). Read the section on gastrulation (p. 47 ff.).

The organizer experiment (Spemann and H. Mangold, 1924) represents the classical case of a complex induction. The authors discovered that the upper lip of the blastopore of a young urodele gastrula, when transplanted to the flank or ventral region of another young gastrula would invaginate, self-differentiate into notochord and somites, and, in addition, induce adjacent host tissue to form a second medullary plate and supplementary mesodermal structures. The self-differentiating transplant and the induced host structures together formed a well-integrated set of "secondary" axial and paraxial structures, with its own polarity and bilateral symmetry, approaching a complete "secondary embryo" at the flank or ventral region of the host embryo. This capacity for integrative inductions has earned the upper lip the designation "organizer." The further analysis was greatly enhanced by the application of "heteroplastic transplantation," i.e., exchange between embryos belonging to two different species, making it possible to distinguish between self-differentiating donor tissue and induced host tissue.

In the organizer action the following components can be distinguished:

1. The transplanted upper lip invaginates. It possesses autonomous gastrulation tendencies.

2. It self-differentiates into notochord and somites or other mesodermal tissue.

3. The transplant induces adjacent host mesoderm to form mesodermal structures, such as contributions to notochord, somites, pronephros, lateral plate, etc. Host and transplant structures supplement each other to form a complete set of mesodermal axial and paraxial organs. The share of the transplant in this secondary set is variable and depends partly on the initial size of the transplant.

4. The transplant induces overlying host ectoderm to form a "secondary" neural tube, which is frequently subdivided into brain with optic vesicles, spinal cord, etc.

In the following, a few points will be discussed which are of importance in planning the experimental work. It was shown that the region of the early gastrula that possesses organizer capacity corresponds to the chordamesoderm area (see map, Fig. 4). Therefore, it is not necessary to use strictly median parts of the upper lip. The results of the experiment differ when dorsal blastopore lips from different stages of gastrulation are used. It will be remembered that the dorsal lip of the early gastrula is composed of material which will come to be head entoderm and mesoderm. The upper lip of late gastrulae is prospective trunk mesoderm. Spemann (1931) has shown that the two differ in their inductive capacities: the head mesoderm has a tendency to induce head structures and is therefore called "head organizer," and the latter, the "trunk organizer," tends to induce trunk structures. It is therefore necessary to check and to record carefully the developmental stage of the donor. However, the host level to which the transplantation is made influences the result. The head-organizer tendencies are strong enough to induce a head in any host level. However, the trunk organizer regularly induces a trunk only in the trunk level, whereas it tends to induce head structures in the head level. In the latter instance the host influence overrides the inherent tendency of the transplant. Since many of the inductions obtained by the student will be partial rather than complete embryos, these findings may help to interpret the results. Finally, the axial orientation of the induced embryo was found to vary considerably; the axes of the host and of the induced embryo may be at any angle with each other. It has been found that the transplant has its intrinsic polarity but that the more powerful gastrulation movements of the host may cause those of the transplant to deviate, so that the final orientation of the induced embryo will be either parallel to the host axis or the resultant between the two tendencies.

The most complete secondary embryos can be obtained when large median pieces of the dorsal lip of early gastrulae are implanted in the ventral lip, opposite to the dorsal lip of the host (Fig. 28, *b*). In this instance, the direction of invagination of the host and of the transplant will be parallel, and host and donor structures will be in corresponding levels. In this way the host will interfere little with the formation of the secondary embryo.

EXPERIMENT 39

Material

gastrulae of *Taricha, Diemictylus*, stages H10–H11 (*Ambystoma* is less suited for this experiment, because the completely decapsulated gastrula is rather flabby and tends to collapse.)

standard equipment (p. 44)

Note.—Use dishes with agar bottom for operations and for raising. Sterilize all instruments carefully.

Procedure

Note.—Since the color differences between donor and host are usually not very striking, the transplant will soon be lost sight of unless it is vital stained. Therefore, vital staining of the donor embryos *in toto* in 0.1 per cent Nile blue sulfate is advisable. Early gastrulae are very delicate when taken out of their membranes, and your success will depend on careful handling and strictly sterile working conditions.

119

1. Select 8–12 healthy gastrulae in the stage of sickle-shaped blastopore (H10½–H10¾). Remove the outer jelly membranes. Wash the embryos (in their vitelline membranes) in dilute medium. Transfer 2 embryos (in a sterile pipette) to an operation dish with concentrated medium.

2. With a sturdy glass needle make 2 rather flat and wide grooves in the agar bottom; they should be close together, so that both embryos are in the visual field. The grooves should be "tailored" to size: They should be somewhat larger in diameter than the gastrulae and not too deep; otherwise, it is difficult to lift the embryos out after the operation. Smooth the edges with a ball tip. Place donor and host in the grooves; they will orient themselves with the animal pole upward because they rotate freely in the perivitelline space. Place several glass bridges in the dish next to the embryos.

3. Remove the vitelline membrane from both embryos. The embryos can now be oriented. Using the hair loop, turn them over with very gentle movements, so that the blastopores face upward.

4. *Prepare the host.*—Of the two embryos, choose as the host the one that

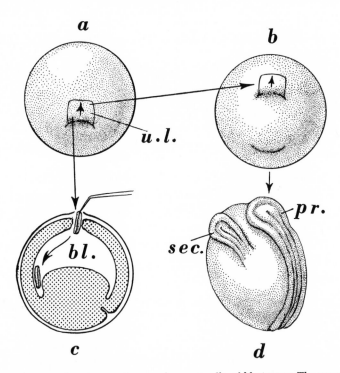

F_IG. 28.—Organizer experiments. a = donor; $u.l.$ = upper lip of blastopore. The arrow indicates the main axis. b = host embryo with its dorsal (upper) lip facing downward; transplant (with arrow, indicating its orientation) in the region of the ventral lip of the host. c = implantation into the blastocoele ($bl.$). d = induction of secondary medullary plate ($sec.$). $pr.$ = medullary plate of host embryo,

120

is less injured. With the tip of a very fine needle cut out a square area of the surface layer opposite to the blastopore, approximately in the region where the ventral lip would appear later. The hole should not be too large or too deep (Fig. 28, *b*). Remove a few of the large yolk cells.

5. *Cut out the transplant*.—Place the donor in such a position that the upper lip points away from you. Cut out a square piece of the upper lip, slightly larger than the hole in the host. Make three cuts and include the upper lip itself as the fourth edge (Fig. 28, *a*). Remove loose entoderm cells on the inner surface with the tip of the glass needle. Do not lose the orientation of the transplant. Use color differences as landmarks.

6. *Implantation*.—Transfer the transplant to the host on the tip of the needle or with the hair loop. Implant in such a way that the dorsal lip of the transplant is opposite to that of the host (Fig. 28, *b*). Press the transplant gently into position, fit it in tightly, and enlarge the hole if necessary. Push the glass bridge over the transplant (with 2 hair loops) and press it down gently so that the transplant fits in well and is in the desired orientation. Remove the donor embryo to another dish. Cover the operation dish at once and shove it gently aside; do not lift it up. Healing takes $\frac{1}{2}$–1 hour. Control the progress of healing but disturb the embryo as little as possible. Readjust the glass bridge if necessary.

7. After 45–60 minutes, cautiously remove the glass bridge. Very cautiously replace the concentrated solution stepwise by dilute medium, using a sterile pipette. Release the fluid very gently; avoid all currents. Remove all debris.

8. Take a careful record; make sketches. Indicate stage, size, shape, and orientation of transplant.

Note.—Make 3–4 operations.

9. During the following days disturb the embryo as little as possible; handle it with utmost care. After gastrulation is complete, turn it right side up to allow neural folds to develop normally. Watch for an induced neural plate. Make sketches.

10. The induced embryo is usually at its best in stages during and after the closure of the neural folds (Fig. 28, *d*) and in earliest tail-bud stages. Study and draw these stages carefully. The early tail-bud stage is a critical stage; from then on mortality is high. Fix in stage H20 or stage H21. If you wish to rear an embryo longer, watch it every few hours for the first signs of disintegration and fix at once. Disintegration proceeds very rapidly, once it has started.

f) IMPLANTATION OF THE ORGANIZER IN THE BLASTOCOELE

Spemann and O. Mangold found that a piece of the organizer when placed in the blastcoele of a blastula will be shifted into the anterior, ventral region of the embryo by the gastrulation movements of the host and will induce a secondary embryo in this position (*Einsteck*-method). In some instances it may be found in other locations. Its final location cannot be determined exactly by the experimenter. This disadvantage, however, is outweighed by the advantages of this technique. It is a much simpler and faster experiment than the transplantation. Furthermore, it makes it possible to test the inductive capacity of structures which cannot be transplanted to the surface of the gastrula, as for instance, adult tissue, killed tissues, or tissue extracts or chemical substances, which can be absorbed in agar and implanted in this way. The rapid progress in the analysis of the chemical nature of the induction process was greatly enhanced by this technical advance.

EXPERIMENT 40

Material

    Ambystoma, any species; stages H10–H11, preferably H10$\frac{1}{2}$ or H10$\frac{3}{4}$, as donors; stages H10–H10$\frac{1}{2}$ as hosts. *Triturus*, *Taricha*, corresponding stages (The latter are preferable to *Ambystoma punctatum*.)

    standard equipment

    Note.—Observe all precautions for sterilization carefully.

Procedure:

1–2. Follow steps 1 and 2 on page 120.

3. *Prepare the transplant.*—Remove the vitelline membrane from the donor gastrula by grasping it with two very fine forceps near the animal pole and tearing it (injury of the animal pole region is immaterial). With the hair loop or platinum wire loop turn the embryo over so that the dorsal blastoporal lip faces you. With the glass needle cut out a sizable piece of the upper blastoporal lip. Make three cuts and let the blastoporal lip be the fourth edge (Fig. 28, *a*). Leave the transplant in position; do not lift it out yet.

4. *Prepare the host.*—Grasp the vitelline membrane at the animal pole with two fine watchmaker forceps. Very cautiously tear a hole in the membrane but DO NOT remove it altogether. A small injury to the roof of the gastrula cannot be avoided. The hole can be used for implantation.

5. *Implantation.*—Lift the transplant from the donor and turn it upside down. With the tip of a fine glass needle or a loop very carefully and gently remove the large spherical entoderm cells which adhere to it. With the glass needle enlarge the slit in the roof of the host gastrula, but do not make it larger than absolutely necessary (Fig. 28, *c*). Lift the transplant with the tip of the needle or the loop on top of the donor. Very gently work it into the hole with the tip of the glass needle. Push the transplant to the ventral side of the blastocoele in a deep position, so that it is out of sight, and very gently pull the edges of the opening together with the tip of the glass needle to facilitate

healing. If the transplant remains near the hole, it may interfere with the healing process or even escape to the outside.

6. After $\frac{1}{2}$–1 hour, replace the concentrated solution stepwise by dilute solution, or pipette embryo very gently into a dish with dilute solution. Longer exposure to concentrated solution may result in exogastrulation (see p. 130). Remove the donor and all debris. Cover the dish and move it gently to a safe place.

7. Take a careful record.

Note.—Make several identical operations.

8. Leave the embryos undisturbed, but check them several times a day. Sometimes the torn vitelline membrane constricts the embryo and interferes with the normal gastrulation process. In this case, remove it completely. After gastrulation is completed, turn the embryo dorsal side up to allow neural folds to develop normally.

9. When neurula stages are reached, watch for induced neural plates and folds. The inductions are usually at their best during and after the closure of the neural folds and in early tail-bud stages. Study and sketch these stages carefully. Only few embryos will survive longer. If you wish to fix and section older embryos, watch them closely every few hours, and fix them when they show the first sign of loss of cells or edema.

Study the papers of Holtfreter (1934 *a, b*) and try to obtain inductions with living or dead tissue of adult salamanders (brain, retina) or with pieces of medullary plate or ectoderm which have been killed by heat or in alcohol (wash carefully before implanting). There is a strong tendency for such implants to be extruded. Healing has to be watched closely. Use species other than *Ambystoma* if possible.

BIBLIOGRAPHY

HOLTFRETER, J. 1934a. Der Einfluss thermischer, mechanischer und chemischer Eingriffe auf die Induzierfähigkeit von Triton-Keimteilen. Arch. f. Entw'mech., **132**:226.

———. 1934b. Über die Verbreitung induzierender Substanzen und ihre Leistungen im Triton-Keim. *Ibid.*, p. 308.

——— and HAMBURGER, V. 1955. Amphibians. In WILLIER, WEISS, and HAMBURGER (eds.), Analysis of development. Philadelphia: Saunders.

SPEMANN, H. 1931. Über den Anteil von Implantat und Wirtskeim an der Orientierung und Beschaffenheit der induzierten Embryonalanlage. Arch. f. Entw'mech., **123**:390.

———. 1938. Embryonic development and induction. New Haven: Yale University Press.

——— and MANGOLD, H. 1924. Über Induktion von Embryonalanlagen durch Implantation artfremder Organisatoren. Arch. f. mikr. Anat. u. Entw'mech., **100**:599.

7. PARABIOSIS

This method consists of the fusion of 2 whole embryos, side by side. This is accomplished by creating wound surfaces in corresponding regions in the flank of 2 embryos and bringing the wounds in apposition to each other. Compression of the embryos facilitates the healing process. Such Siamese-type twins can be reared to metamorphosis. (*Note.*—True Siamese twins originate from one egg, by incomplete separation of its two halves; see p. 79.)

This method has been found useful for several purposes. It can be used for "nursing" of experimental embryos that would otherwise not be capable of surviving. For instance, embryos in which essential parts of the nervous system have been removed can be reared by uniting them with a normal embryo. A fruitful application of the method has been in the field of physiology of sex determination. Conjoined twins share a common blood circulation, and their sex hormones are distributed to both partners. Since 50 per cent of the parabiotic twins are expected to be male-female combinations, valuable material can thus be obtained for the study of the interaction between genetic and hormonal sex determiners. Burns (since 1925; see 1955) and Witschi (1934, 1939) have applied this technique extensively. Witschi has also used an end-to-end fusion (telobiosis).

EXPERIMENT 41

Material

> urodele larvae, stages H22–H27; anuran larvae, stage PM16
> standard equipment (p. 44)
> steel needle with sharp edge, in needle holder
> operation dishes with bottom of beeswax.

Prepare small glass blocks to hold the embryos in position during fusion. With the diamond pencil, scratch a grid of squares, 4–5 mm.^{2} on a clean microscope slide. Break the square pieces apart; if necessary use a pair of forceps with broad prongs. Hold the edges of each square in the flame of the microburner until they are completely smooth. Prepare 6–10 blocks and keep them in a clean covered dish.

Procedure (Fig. 29)

1. Select a number of healthy embryos of identical stage; remove all membranes. Keep them in dilute medium; cover the dish.

2. In the operation dish prepare with a ball tip a shallow groove in which the embryo fits when placed right or left side up. At some distance, prepare a deep rectangular groove with vertical walls, using the steel needle. The groove should be slightly narrower than the greatest width of the two embryos and not much longer than the embryos; otherwise they may slip out. It should be so deep that the embryos are almost buried when placed in it, dorsal side down. Their bellies should be flush with the surface or extending slightly above it. Smooth the walls and bottom of the groove carefully with a small ball tip to avoid injury to the embryos. Place two embryos in the groove before you start

124

operations and make sure that the groove fits tightly; this is very important for the success of the experiment. Place several glass blocks in the dish.

3. With the glass needle cut out a rather large circular or square area of ectoderm from the left flank of one embryo and from the right flank of the other (Fig. 29, *a*). Operate behind the gill swelling, rather far dorsally. Make the wounds as nearly identical in size and topographic region as possible.

4. Immediately after the wounds have been prepared, place the two embryos in the groove, with the dorsal sides down and the wounds in apposition. The wounds must be pressed together tightly. Ciliary movement may be disturbing. Hold the embryos in position with a glass block. The weight may compress the bellies slightly, but not too much. Allow sufficient time for com-

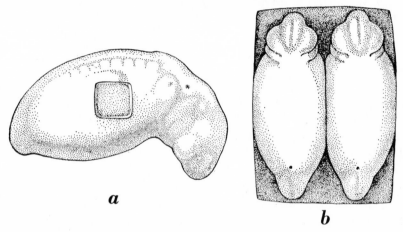

a

b

Fig. 29.—Parabiosis of two urodele embryos. *a* = removal of part of flank epidermis; *b* = the two embryos placed in rectangular groove in beeswax.

plete fusion; this may take several hours. The embryos fall apart easily if they are not well healed together. Very cautiously shift the glass weight to the side and lift the pair out of the groove; if necessary, cut out one wall of the groove with the steel needle.

4*a*. An alternative method uses the *glass blocks* to hold the embryos together. Smooth the edges carefully in the microburner. Prepare a shallow groove in the wax with straight walls; place the embryos in it, dorsal side down, and the wounds in apposition. Place 1 block on each side of the groove and lean the embryos against them. Carefully and gently push the two blocks against the embryos, one at a time, until the embryos are slightly compressed. Make sure that the wound surfaces are pressed against each other. Place a glass bridge on top of the embryos if necessary.

5. When the pair is firmly fused after several hours, or overnight, transfer them to a glass dish or paraffined paper cup in dilute medium. Use a wide-

mouthed pipette and handle the embryos very gently. Avoid squirting and water currents.

6. Observe the development of the pair, their heart beat, swimming movements, etc. Start feeding them at the appropriate time (see p. 26). Sectioning is necessary for the study of the gonads.

BIBLIOGRAPHY

BURNS, R. K. JR. 1925. The sex of parabiotic twins in Amphibia. Jour. Exper. Zool., **42**:31.
———. 1955. Urogenital system. In WILLIER, WEISS, and HAMBURGER (eds.), Analysis of development. Philadelphia: Saunders.
WITSCHI, E. 1934. Genes and inductors of sex differentiation in amphibians. Quart. Rev. Biol., **9**:460.
———. 1939. Modification of the development of sex in lower vertebrates and in mammals. In ALLEN, E., *et al.*, Sex and internal secretions. Baltimore: Williams & Wilkins.

8. EXTRINSIC FACTORS IN DEVELOPMENT

a) INTRODUCTORY REMARKS

Embryos can adjust to considerable variations in their environment. What we designate as their "normal" milieu is the range of conditions (characteristic for each species) that permits normal development. Excessive changes, beyond these limits, in such factors as temperature, chemical composition of the medium, etc., result in developmental abnormalities. Since many external agents permit a quantitative approach, they have become a valuable tool in the hands of the experimental embryologist. Furthermore, the experimental analysis of abnormalities produced in this way has been helpful in an understanding of the great variety of naturally occurring and hereditary malformations in animals and man.

Two broad generalizations have been deduced from investigations of this kind: (1) The same agent can produce a number of different effects, depending on dosage, duration of application, and stage of development at which it is applied. (2) Similar or identical effects can often be produced by entirely different agents. These findings have led to the notion that the different embryonic areas or developmental processes pass through "sensitive periods" during which they are particularly susceptible to a variety of deleterious agents, and it seems that the pattern of these "differential susceptibilities" plays a more important role in determining the end effect than the nature of the extrinsic agent itself.

Of the large body of material which could be used to illustrate these and other principles, two representative experiments were selected. They concern the effects of changes in the chemical composition of the medium on amphibian development. Experiments dealing with other extrinsic agents, such as temperature, oxygen tension, dietary factors, or irradiation experiments with ultraviolet or X-rays, can be designed by the instructor, depending on available special equipment.

b) LITHIUM EXPERIMENTS

The peculiar effects of LiCl on early development were discovered by C. Herbst (1893) in his pioneer study of the effects of changes in the ionic composition of the medium on sea-urchin development. He found that when early stages are reared in sea water to which a low concentration of LiCl has been added, part of the material destined to become ectoderm is "entodermized," resulting in a disproportionately large inestine that evaginates during gastrulation instead of invaginating, thus forming an "exogastrula."

Exposure of early amphibian embryos to high concentrations of LiCl (1 per cent) results likewise in exogastrulation (see p. 130). If lower concentrations (of approximately 0.5–0.8 per cent) are applied to blastulae and gastrulae for periods of 5–24 hours, a variety of abnormalities results, the most conspicuous feature being an underdevelopment ("hypomorphosis") of head structures (Adelmann, 1936; Hall, 1942; Lehmann, 1945; Pasteels, 1945; and others). Not only is the head disproportionately small ("microcephaly"), but its bilateral structures, such as suckers or balancers, nasal pits, eyes, show varying degrees of approximation toward the median plane. Microscopic studies show that the internal head structures, such as the visceral arches and the pharynx, are also affected. In more extreme cases only a single unpaired structure may be found in or near the mid-line. The appearance of single median nasal pits is referred to as "monorhyny," that of single median eyes as "cyclopia," and that of single ear vesicles as "otocephaly." In a further step of reduction, the greater part of the head may be suppressed altogether. Finally, the deficiencies may extend to the trunk and tail, including spina bifida (local failure of spinal canal and spinal cord to close), edema, and scoliosis (lateral curvature of the axis).

In performing the experiment outlined below, the student will find considerable individual variations in the same experimental lot. A study of these variations, as well as a comparison of the types of hypomorphoses obtained in different experiments, is instructive. It may not be possible to arrange the abnormalities in a linear order of degrees of severity, because different parts of the complex head may vary independently of one another. Yet they all follow a definite pattern: As a rule, the more median parts are more severely affected than the more lateral parts, and the anterior parts more severely than the posterior parts. Generally speaking, one recognizes a medio-lateral and an anterior-posterior *gradient*[15] of susceptibility. Obviously the lithium treatment

---

[15] The significance of gradients of susceptibility in the origin of developmental abnormalities and the general role of physiological gradients in development has been stressed particularly by C. M. Child (see 1941; see also p. 178 below).

127

does not affect individual organ primordia or their precursors; rather, it modifies and distorts the *over-all pattern of head formation*.

Similar types of hypomorphoses of the head can be produced by other agents, such as $MgCl_2$ or high temperature. In this connection, it is of interest to note that abnormalities, such as microcephaly or cyclopia, are not uncommon among other vertebrates and man. They occur either "spontaneously" (that is, from unknown causes), or as the result of different experimental procedures, or as mutants. All these observations illustrate the notion of "differential susceptibility." In all vertebrates the process of determination of head structures seems to pass through a critical "sensitive period" during which it is vulnerable to a variety of quite unrelated deleterious agencies.

It would be misleading, however, to make a sharp distinction between "nonspecific" external agents and "specific" intrinsic developmental patterns. Taking a physiological viewpoint, one must assume that each extrinsic agent exerts its inhibitory or retarding action on a particular metabolic step or a particular structural element in the cell. Considerable work has been devoted to the study of the effects of LiCl on cell metabolism and cell structure; (review in Gustafson, 1950; for amphibians see Lallier, 1954), but the primary action of the Li ion is not yet elucidated. The principle that different agents may nevertheless produce the same abnormalities is readily understood if one realizes that each agent may interfere with a different link in the chain of events leading to the terminal state. Altogether the term "specific" is ambiguous in this context and should be avoided. In the final analysis, embryonic differentiation is the result of a complex, delicately balanced interplay of extrinsic and intrinsic factors and conditions, and the processes involved in the determination of head structures, or of any other pattern or structure, can be thrown out of gear vicariously by "intrinsic" factors, such as mutant gene products, or by non-physiological "extrinsic" agents, such as lithium salts.

The Li experiments can be used to good advantage as an exercise in experimental design. Since the embryos respond sensitively to slight differences in the treatment, one can set up a number of parallel experiments in each of which one factor is varied and all others kept constant. Variations in stage of development, dosage, and temperature are easy to manipulate; students can work in teams, each team exploring a different variable. It should be realized that different batches of eggs may differ slightly in their responses and that experimental results are therefore not always reproducible. However, it is not difficult to obtain a series of effects, ranging from slight hypomorphoses of the head all the way to exogastrulation.

The experiment described below is a standard experiment which was selected because it gave rather consistently typical hypomorphoses of the head (in *Rana pipiens*).

Material

    late blastulae or early gastrulae of *Rana pipiens*

    glass jars or finger bowls

    pipettes

    lithium chloride, c.p., 0.8 per cent in distilled water

Note.—The following data apply to *Rana pipiens*. The optimal experimental conditions for obtaining similar hypomorphoses in other species should be determined in advance by the instructor. If you find exogastrulae, consult page 130. If possible, use a constant-temperature room or refrigerator (between 15° and 24° C.). Otherwise keep a record of the room temperature.

Procedure

    1. Under the binocular microscope remove all membranes, except the vitelline membrane, from 50–60 eggs, using watchmaker forceps.

    2. Place 25–30 embryos in a finger bowl containing 0.8 per cent LiCl and an equal number in boiled tap water or dilute medium, as controls. In pipetting the experimental embryos avoid diluting the LiCl solution.

    3. After 5 hours remove the embryos from the LiCl solution, wash them in a large amount of boiled tap water or dilute medium, and rear them in this medium. Take a careful record of dosage, stage at exposure, time of exposure, temperature. Label all dishes carefully.

    4. Observe the further development. Note and sketch the first deviations from normal development by comparing with controls. Watch particularly the dislocation of suckers and nasal pits toward the mid-line, and shape and size of the head.

    5. Allow the animals to develop until the cornea is transparent and the pigmented eyes are clearly visible (approximately stage 24 or stage 25). Narcotize all embryos, place them side by side with normal embryos, and study the different degrees of head hypomorphosis. Pay special attention to suckers, nasal pits, eyes. Try to arrange the abnormalities in a graded series of degrees of hypomorphosis and tabulate them. Fix all embryos, including some normal controls, in 10 per cent formaldehyde. After thorough fixation, dissect the most interesting cases with forceps and strong glass needles. Carefully remove the skin over the head. Notice reduction in size of brain, size and position of eyes, etc.

Note.—Perform several parallel series of experiments, following the suggestions given above.

BIBLIOGRAPHY

ADELMANN, H. B. 1936. The problem of cyclopia. Quart. Rev. Biol., **11:**161, 284.

CHILD, C. M. 1941. Patterns and problems of development. Chicago: University of Chicago Press.

Gustafson, T. 1950. Survey of the morphogenetic action of the lithium ion and the chemical basis of its action. Rev. Suisse de Zool., **57** (Suppl. 1) : 77.

Hall, T. S. 1942. The mode of action of lithium salts in amphibian development. Jour. Exper. Zool., **89**:1.

Herbst, C. 1893. Weiteres über die morphologische Wirkung der Lithium-Salze. Mitt. zool. Stat. Neapel, **11**:136.

Lallier, R. 1954. Chlorure de lithium et biochimie du développement de l'œuf d'Amphibien. Jour. Embryol. & Exper. Morphol., **2**:323.

Lehmann, F. E. 1945. Einführung in die physiologische Embryologie, pp. 304 ff. Basel: Birkhauser.

Pasteels, J. 1945. Recherches sur l'action du LiCl sur les œufs des Amphibiens. Arch. de biol., **56**:105.

c) EXOGASTRULATION AND SPINA BIFIDA PRODUCED BY TREATMENT WITH HYPERTONIC SALT SOLUTION

Before starting this experiment the student should familiarize himself with the normal gastrulation movements (pp. 47 ff.). Exogastrulation is a disturbance of the gastrulation process: Mesoderm and endoderm fail to invaginate under the ectodermal covering; they remain outside but continue their typical gastrulation movements in the opposite direction and move away from the ectoderm, from which they become gradually separated by a constriction (Fig. 30)

Exogastrulation is a rather common abnormality of early development found in many forms. It can be produced experimentally in amphibians by a variety of changes of the culture medium, such as exposure to a hypertonic salt solution or to high, sublethal concentrations of lithium chloride or magnesium chloride. The most extensive analysis was done by Holtfreter (1933a, b), who exposed urodele embryos to his "standard" solution (concentrated Holtfreter solution), from the blastula stage on. He followed the exogastrulation movements by vital-stain markings and succeeded in rearing some exogastrulae to advanced stages. He obtained a graded series of exogastrulae. In total exogastrulation, the ectoderm is separated almost completely from the endoderm and mesoderm. The latter proceed surprisingly far in their differentiation, in spite of the absence of the ectodermal covering and in spite of the complete inversion of all structures (endoderm outside, mesoderm inside); however, the ectodermal vesicle fails to undergo any differentiation (Fig. 30, b). In partial exogastrulation, the mesoderm and endoderm invaginate in varying degrees, resulting in partial embryos (see Holtfreter, 1933b, for urodeles; Holtfreter and Hamburger, 1955, Fig. 79, for anurans). In all instances, only that part of the ectoderm that is underlain by invaginated mesoderm differentiates into neural tube, sense organs, and other ectodermal derivatives. This finding, together with the complete lack of differentiation of the ectoderm in total exogastrulae strongly supports the notion that mesodermal induction is necessary for neural differentiation. In the least affected cases, the yolk plug merely fails to move inside; it blocks the fusion of the medullary folds locally. In later stages, this deficiency appears as a slit in the spinal cord known as "spina bifida" (Fig. 30, c, d).

Experiment 43

Material

    Ambystoma, any species, stages H7–H9 (The experiment is unsuccessful, if early gastrulae are used.) *Rana,* stages Sh8–9 (Urodele embryos are preferable.)

operation dishes with lids

pipettes

concentrated and dilute culture medium

Note.—Work under strictly sterile conditions.

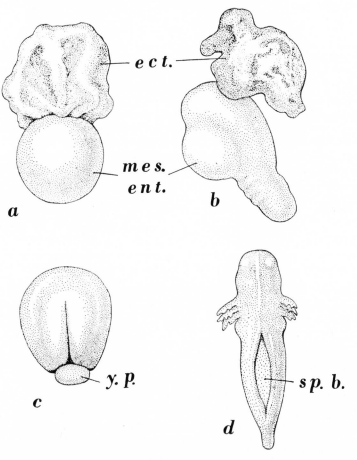

Fig. 30.—Total (*a, b*) and partial exogastrulation (*c, d*) in urodeles (modified after Holtfreter, 1933). *a =* at end of gastrulation; *b =* in early tail-bud stage; *ect. =* ectoderm (undifferentiated); *mes. ent. =* mesodermal and entodermal components. *c =* neurula with incompletely invaginated yolk plug (*y.p.*); *d =* embryo with spina bifida (*sp. b.*).

131

Procedure

1. Remove the outer membranes from 20 to 30 embryos. Although the removal of the vitelline membrane enhances exogastrulation, it is recommended that it be left intact, because it is difficult to remove it in these early stages.

2. Place 15–20 embryos in concentrated solution in several agar dishes, and the remainder in dilute medium, as controls. Observe the process of exogastrulation during the following days. Various degrees of exogastrulation will be noticed. Make sketches of representative cases. Discard dying embryos and all debris.

3. Raise the embryos as long as possible. Notice ectodermal differentiation in partial exogastrulae and the wrinkled appearance of undifferentiated ectoderm that is not underlain by mesoderm. Notice "spina bifida" in the least affected cases.

Note.—The range of variations can be increased by using slightly higher or slightly lower concentrations of the culture medium.

BIBLIOGRAPHY

HOLTFRETER, J. 1933*a*. Die totale Exogastrulation, eine Selbstablösung des Ektoderms vom Entomesoderm. Entwicklung und funktionelles Verhalten nervenloser Organe. Arch. f. Entw'mech., **129**:669.

———. 1933*b*. Organisierungsstufen nach regionaler Kombination von Entomesoderm mit Ektoderm. Biol. Zentralbl., **53**:404.

——— and HAMBURGER, V. 1955. Amphibians. In WILLIER, WEISS, and HAMBURGER (eds.), Analysis of development. Philadelphia: Saunders.

9. HORMONAL CONTROL OF METAMORPHOSIS IN *AMPHIBIA*[16]

a) INTRODUCTORY REMARKS

The larvae of some animal groups are highly specialized in adaptation to a mode of life different from that of the adult. In such forms, the transformation from one state to the other involves a sequence of radical and often rapid changes in structural and functional characters, referred to as "metamorphosis." In the two groups which are most readily accessible to the experimental analysis of this phenomenon, insects and amphibians, metamorphosis was found to be controlled by hormones. In amphibians, the thyroid gland produces a hormone which controls metamorphosis. Its most active fraction, the amino acid *thyroxin* (containing 65 per cent of iodine), has been synthesized and is available in crystalline form. The thyroid gland, in turn, is under the control of the thyrotropic hormone, secreted by the anterior lobe of the hypophysis.

Ever since Gudernatsch (1912) discovered that the metamorphosis of tadpoles can be precipitated by the feeding of thyroid gland, the mechanism of its action has been investigated extensively by a number of experimental proce-

[16] I am indebted to Drs. W. Etkin and J. Kollros for help and advice in preparing this outline.

dures, such as extirpation of the thyroid primordium in embryos, injection and feeding of thyroid preparations, or immersion of larvae in dilute solutions of such substances (reviews by Lynn and Wachowski, 1951; Etkin, 1955). We have selected one representative experiment as an introduction to this field. Additional experiments suitable for classwork may be found in Adams (1941) and Rugh (1948).

Experimental workers usually distinguish two periods in the over-all process of metamorphosis: The "prometamorphic period," beginning with early stages of the formation of toes in the hind limbs, is characterized mainly by rapid growth of the hind limbs. The "metamorphic climax" that follows is a short period involving more spectacular changes, including emergence of the fore-limbs and the resorption of the tail. Description of the structural changes and timetables of metamorphic events for American frogs may be found in Etkin (1932, 1955) and Taylor and Kollros (1946).

Following is a list of the readily observable structural changes, arranged approximately in the order of their appearance (after Etkin).

1. Rapid growth of hind limbs
2. Resorption of the anal canal, which is the exterior terminal part of the intestinal tract, between the hind legs
3. Thinning of the skin and formation of windows in the gill region, through which the forelimbs emerge
4. Shedding of the horny teeth and beaks and resorption of the lips
5. Emergence of forelimbs; the left, emerging through the widened spiracle, usually appears first
6. Marked growth of eyes
7. Broadening of the mouth
8. Resorption of the tail (begins about simultaneously with 5)
9. First skin shedding
10. Formation of the tympanum

Another change, a loss of water (desiccation) is very pronounced during climax. At the same time, the intestinal contents are evacuated. The resulting shrinkage changes the oval contour of the tadpole to an angular shape. In thy-roxin-treated animals this shrinkage is one of the first and clearest signs of the effectiveness of the treatment. To observe internal changes, such as the marked shortening of the coiled tadpole intestine, specimens in different stages of meta-morphosis have to be dissected. Altogether, this survey shows that metamor-phosis combines growth and differentiation processes in some structures with dedifferentiation and resorption processes in others.

To guarantee a smooth transition from the functional state of the larva to that of the postmetamorphic frog, the partial events of metamorphosis have to be carefully synchronized and integrated. For instance, the shift in loco-motion requires that the resorption of the tail occurs only after the hind limbs have grown and the forelimbs have emerged. This time pattern of metamorphic events is regulated by the thyroid hormone.

How is this accomplished? According to Etkin (1935, 1955), two variables are attuned to each other: the changing hormone concentration in the blood and differential susceptibilities of different structures to a given hormone concentration. Hind legs are the most sensitive structures, whereas the tail belongs to the group of less sensitive organs. In the early prometamorphic period the hormone level in the blood is low, but sufficient to elicit an accelerated growth of the hind legs. Gradually the hormone concentration builds up and attains a peak at "climax." The tail and other less sensitive structures require these high concentrations to give their typical, rapid response. The situation is further complicated by changes in thresholds with progression of differentiation.

It is on the basis of these notions that the experimental results have to be explained. The administration of a relatively high dosage of thyroxin to prometamorphic tadpoles results in the disruption of the normal timetable and a distortion of the normal metamorphic pattern. The increased thyroxin level activates the less sensitive structures precociously and precipitates a "climax" within a few days or a week, depending on the experimental conditions. With high concentrations the onset of climax is so rapid that it does not permit sufficient time for the extensive development of the hind limbs which normally precedes it; hence, shrinkage, tail resorption, shedding of the horny mouth implements, and other changes may occur while the hind legs have advanced only slightly. With lower concentrations, metamorphosis is accelerated but less distorted. Generally speaking, the metamorphic changes in different structures are speeded up at different rates, depending on the relative sensitivity of each structure, and the synchronization of events breaks down. This is evident when the sequence of events in experimental animals is compared with the normal timetable given above and by Etkin (1932, 1955). In addition, truly abnormal features may be observed under certain experimental conditions, such as deformities in the jaws and excessive enlargement of the windows for emergence of the forelegs. Altogether, it is not surprising that few experimental animals survive to the end of metamorphosis.

b) REARING OF TADPOLES IN THYROXIN SOLUTION

EXPERIMENT 44

It is suggested that before the experimental work is started a demonstration be given of representative stages of normal metamorphosis.
Material
    anuran tadpoles, any stage from cone-shaped hind-limb buds to paddle-
      shaped hind limbs (stages III–X, Taylor and Kollros (1946)

large finger bowls for rearing tadpoles (15–20 in each), or small finger
  bowls for 1–3 specimens
Syracuse dishes or casters with cotton, for observation
large pipettes, sieves, or perforated spoons to transfer tadpoles
canned spinach (see p. 27)
10 per cent formaldehyde
thyroxin tablets or dl-thyroxin crystals. Prepare a stock solution of 1:10,000
  made basic by addition of 1 drop of 10 per cent NaOH in 1 cc. of water.
  Keep this stock solution in the refrigerator. Before the start of the experiment, prepare from the stock solution the following dilutions:

$$1:5,000,000 \quad (200 \text{ micrograms/liter})$$
$$1:50,000,000 \quad (20 \text{ micrograms/liter})$$
$$1:100,000,000 \quad (10 \text{ micrograms/liter})$$

Note.—The following data refer to *Rana pipiens*.

Concerning narcosis.—Anuran tadpoles, particularly in prometamorphic
stages, are more sensitive to MS 222 than *Ambystoma* larvae. A concentration
of 1:12,000 can be tolerated for short periods. We recommend that narcosis
not be used but that tadpoles be placed on a pad of thoroughly moistened cotton for observation. All surfaces in contact with the tadpoles must be wet.
Carefully avoid drying. Tadpoles are very sensitive; *avoid all excess handling*
of animals. All instruments and glassware used for fixation must be kept away
from the living animals.

Procedure

1. Select 20 tadpoles of approximately equal size and stage for each experiment, and the same number for controls. For measuring, place them in an open
Petri dish (moist but without excess water) under which a piece of ruled graph
paper has been placed. For staging, place them on a pad of moist cotton.

2. Fill each of 3 large ($7\frac{1}{2}$ in.) finger bowls with 2,000 cc. of one of the thyroxin concentrations listed above, and one with 2,000 cc. boiled tap water.
Mark each dish clearly. Place 20 tadpoles in each dish. Record carefully: date,
concentration, stage, temperature.

3. Change the thyroxin solutions every day. Stop feeding the tadpoles after
the first signs of metamorphosis have appeared. For daily observations, place
one experimental animal and one control at a time, side by side, on a pad of
moist cotton. Make careful observations of the metamorphic changes listed
above and make sketches. Note the differences in the different concentrations.
In our experiments, animals in 1:5,000,000 (at room temperature) showed the
first changes after 2–3 days and survived for 5 days; animals in 1:50,000,000
survived for 7–9 days; animals in 1:100,000,000 showed changes after 4 days
and survived for 2 weeks.

4. Fix dying and dead specimens together with controls in 10 per cent formaldehyde. After 2 or 3 weeks terminate all experiments; fix all survivors and

controls. Dissect different stages; note changes in intestine and other viscera. If you wish to rear specimens through metamorphosis, place them in a finger bowl in which water is shallow enough to prevent drowning of newly metamorphosed animals, or make a slope of sand rising above water level on one side of the finger bowl (see p. 26). Cover the finger bowl with a glass plate. Tabulate your results and write a brief summary, indicating the sequence of events and the abnormal features. Compare the results obtained in different thyroxin concentrations.

BIBLIOGRAPHY

ADAMS, A. E. 1941. Studies in experimental zoology. 2d ed. Ann Arbor: Edwards Brothers.
ETKIN, W. 1932. Growth and resorption phenomena in anuran metamorphosis. I. Physiol. Zoöl., **5**:275.
———. 1935. The mechanisms of anuran metamorphosis. I. Jour. Exper. Zool., **71**:317.
———. 1955. Metamorphosis. In WILLIER, WEISS, and HAMBURGER (eds.), Analysis of development. Philadelphia: Saunders.
GUDERNATSCH, J. F. 1912. Feeding experiments on tadpoles. I. Roux' Arch. Entw'mech., **35**:457.
LYNN, W. G., and WACHOWSKI, H. 1951. The thyroid gland and its functions in cold-blooded vertebrates. Quart. Rev. Biol., **26**:123.
RUGH, ROBERTS. 1948. Experimental Embryology: A Manual of Techniques and Procedures. Minneapolis: Burgess Pub. Co.
TAYLOR, A. C., and KOLLROS, J. J. 1946. Stages in the normal development of *Rana pipiens* larvae. Anat. Rec., **94**:7.

10. THE DEVELOPMENT OF BEHAVIOR PATTERNS

a) THE ORIGIN OF EARLY REFLEXES

Behavior patterns, like organs, have an ontogenetic development. The development of behavior is studied best in the reflexes of lower vertebrate embryos. The classical work of G. E. Coghill on the early reflexes of salamander larvae has led him to far-reaching conclusions. Some of his observations on *Ambystoma* larvae can easily be repeated and are therefore introduced here. His book, *Anatomy and the Problem of Behavior* (1929), should be consulted in connection with this exercise.

Swimming is the first integrated activity of an amphibian larva. Its origin was studied by Coghill with his interest focused on the problem: Is this reflex the result of "learning," or is it entirely the result of the maturation of the nervous system, with no contribution from "experience"?

Swimming is preceded by spontaneous wriggling motions within the membranes, long before hatching. Coghill studied in detail these earliest movements in *Ambystoma punctatum* and classified them in a number of behavior stages (p. 138). This series shows clearly the progression in the complexity of the behavior pattern. A slight bending of the head is the first perceptible movement. It is followed by a more intense bend, or coil, extending from the head tailward. The addition of a second coil in the opposite direction before the first has reached the tail results in an S-like wriggle; the swimming emerges from this double flexure as a series of continuous and more powerful S-reactions. Coghill succeeded in accounting for each step in this behavior development in terms of a stepwise increase in the complexity of the nervous system. With each stage a new type of neuron, or connection, is added. The following experiments and observations obtain their full significance only in the light of these neurological data. The student should study the diagrams of the organization of the nervous system in different stages of behavior (in Coghill, 1929).

The general conclusions at which Coghill arrived have influenced considerably our concepts concerning the origin of behavior and of reflexes. In contradiction to the views held by many psychologists and biologists, he demonstrated, at least for his object, that complex behavior patterns do not originate by assembling separate simple reflexes and integrating them secondarily but that the reverse is true: all activities are integrated first, and each step emerges from the preceding one as an integrated unit. Local reflexes are secondarily emancipated from an integrated total pattern by a process called "individuation." The origin of the swimming reflex illustrates this principle. The origin of independent limb movements is another example. To quote Coghill:

The first movement of the fore limb is adduction and abduction. When this movement of the limb is first performed it occurs only with trunk movement. When the trunk acts vigorously, as in swimming, the fore limbs are drawn close against the body. . . .
A day or two ordinarily elapses between the time when the arm begins to move with the action of the trunk before it acquires the ability to respond to a local stimulus without the perceptible action of the trunk. . . . It is obvious, therefore, that the first limb movement is an integral part of the total reaction of the animal, and that it is only later that the limb acquires an individuality of its own in behavior [1929, pp. 18 f.].

The same individuation was observed in jaw movements in feeding, gill movements, etc. However, the progression from integrated to individuated responses is perhaps not so universal a phenomenon as Coghill thought. Coghill worked mainly on *Ambystoma punctatum*. In other urodeles, such as the *Axolotl* and *Triturus taeniatus*, the first limb movements were observed to occur independently of trunk movements (Faber, 1956). The early behavior of mammalian fetuses does not follow a uniform pattern either (Hooker, 1952).

It is necessary to make a clear distinction between this problem of the sequence of events in early behavior and the question, raised above, concerning the role of "trial and error" and "experience" in the origin of integrated behavior. Whereas generalizations with respect to the former are premature, the answer to the latter is clear: Complex performances, such as swimming, walking, and snapping for food, originate as the result of an orderly sequence of events in the maturation of the central nervous system and not as the result of "trial and error." However, experience and learning may improve such patterns as soon as they have come into existence.

137

These stages were worked out by Coghill. The following definitions are taken from DuShane and Hutchinson (1941, pp. 250–51), with a few additions:

NR: Premotile Stage.—No response to repeated touch and deep pressure on the myotomes.

NM: The nonmotile or myotomic response.—This occurs in the absence of, and earlier than, the "early flexure." It is characteristically a slow contraction toward the side stimulated, followed by a slow relaxation. It begins with a bending of the head. This is regarded as a direct non-nervous response of the myotomes.

EF: The early-flexure response.—This is a rather rapid reflex response of the animal to gentle touch. The bending of the body, beginning at the head, is always away from the side stimulated (contralateral). The reaction is brief in duration, the relaxation being abrupt. With further development of the myotomes and the nervous system, the contracted phase tends to be held for a longer period of time and the tail is brought progressively nearer the head. There is no sharp natural distinction between the more advanced flexures and the next stage.

Coil.—The coil reaction is aptly named. It is the culmination of the early flexure and is attained when the tail touches or passes the head at the height of the response. It is again away from the stimulated side (i.e., contralateral). Some embryos show the coil reaction in typical fashion, followed by a coil in the opposite direction without additional external stimulation.

S-reaction.—This is a reaction superimposed upon the coil reaction. It results when a wave of contraction passes down the stimulated side before the original contralateral contraction has relaxed. The embryo is transitorily in the form of the letter S. Occasionally, in response to a single touch the reaction may be repeated several times successively, but it does not yet result in locomotion.

ES: The early-swimming response.—Repeated S-reactions become so organized and strengthened that the embryo makes some forward progress. Embryos that show any progression not more than approximately 3 body lengths fall into this category.

SS: Strong swimmers.—Embryos that swim for more than 3 body lengths to less than 10 body lengths.

LS: Late swimmers.—Embryos that swim 10 or more lengths.

EXPERIMENT 45: OBSERVATIONS ON THE EARLIEST REFLEXES OF *Ambystoma* LARVAE

Material

embryos of *Ambystoma punctatum* in all stages from H31 to H46
glass dishes
a hair loop or a fine hair or bristle mounted in a glass handle

Procedure

Choose embryos of different stages. Place one after another in a dish. Make all observations under the binocular dissecting microscope. With the hair loop stroke the embryo gently along the row of the right myotomes. Observe the reaction as carefully as possible. Take a record of the reaction in terms of the behavior stages listed above and of the Harrison stages. Repeat these observations on a considerable number of embryos and find representative specimens for each Coghill stage. Tabulate your observations in a correlation table. You will observe that there is some variation of behavior reactions in embryos of the same Harrison stage. For instance, embryos in stage H35 may exhibit any of the following reflex responses: NM, EF, Coil, S. Such variations may be found even in material from the same lot of eggs. DuShane and Hutchinson (1941) have devoted a special investigation to this variability. They have given precise data for the range of variation of behavior stages in terms of Harrison stages for two different temperatures. The results of the class should be compiled and compared with Table 1 and Figure 1 of the paper quoted above.

b) DEVELOPMENT OF REFLEX ACTIVITY IN NARCOTIZED EMBRYOS

It is possible to give experimental evidence for the contention that "learning" plays no role in the formation of the swimming reflex. In connection with another study, Harrison (1904) placed frog embryos of early tail-bud stages, i.e., previous to the first movements, in chloretone and kept them in a narcotized condition for as long as 7 days. They were returned to normal water at a stage when the controls were swimming larvae. After a short period of recovery they began to swim normally. Obviously, the nervous system and also the musculature had developed normally in complete absence of functional activity. Later experiments along similar lines have shown that we are dealing here with a general principle of development that holds for organs and structures as well as for the ontogeny of behavior. Most structures, such as the eye or the kidney, are differentiated first and begin to function later.

The narcotization experiments of Harrison were repeated on *Ambystoma* embryos by Matthews and Detwiler (1926). The following experiment is based on this paper, which should be consulted for details.

EXPERIMENT 46

Material

Ambystoma, any species, stage H28 or stage H29

Petri dishes or section dishes with tightly fitting lids

chloretone 1:3,000 or MS 222, between 1:5,000 and 1:6,000; dilute culture medium

hair loop

139

Note.—The mortality in narcotics is high. Different batches of eggs may require different concentrations. The appropriate concentration should be tested in advance.

Procedure

1. Select 15 healthy embryos in a stage preceding the onset of muscular movements (H28 or H29). Remove all membranes. Place 10 specimens in a dish with one of the narcotics mentioned above; keep 5 embryos in dilute medium as controls. Cover both dishes.

2. During the following week change the narcotic daily; keep the dishes tightly covered to prevent evaporation; remove dead animals. By gently stroking the narcotized animals with the hair loop, check each day to see that they are completely immobilized. If not, transfer them to a stronger concentration.

3. When the embryos have reached stages H38–H40 and the controls are swimming larvae, transfer the narcotized embryos to dilute medium. Watch their recovery. Stimulate with the hair loop. Take notes.

BIBLIOGRAPHY (*a–b*)

COGHILL, G. E. 1929. Anatomy and the problem of behaviour. Cambridge, England: Cambridge University Press.

DuSHANE, G. P., and HUTCHINSON, C. 1941. The effect of temperature on the development of form and behavior in amphibian embryos. Jour. Exper. Zool., **87**:245.

FABER, J. 1956. The development and coordination of larval limb movements in *Triturus taeniatus* and *Ambystoma Mexicanum*. Arch. Ne'erl. de Zool., **11**:498.

HARRISON, R. G. 1904. An experimental study of the relation of the nervous system to the developing musculature in the embryo of the frog. Amer. Jour. Anat., **3**:197.

HOOKER, D. 1952. The prenatal origin of behavior. Lawrence: University of Kansas Press.

MATTHEWS, S. A., and DETWILER, S. R. 1926. The reactions of *Amblystoma* embryos following prolonged treatment with chloretone. Jour. Exper. Zool., **45**:279.

PART III
EXPERIMENTS ON THE CHICK EMBRYO

A. MATERIAL AND EQUIPMENT

1. LIVING MATERIAL: INCUBATION

The chick embryo ranks second to the amphibian embryo as a material for the experimental analysis of embryonic development. During the past decades the classical methods of extirpation, transplantation, explantation, and vital staining have been applied successfully to the chick. In addition, the method of chorio-allantoic grafting has given valuable information concerning the potencies of early primordia. The availability of eggs at almost any time of the year and the short duration of early development are great advantages in experimental work with this form.

Data on different breeds, on the principles and practice of incubation, on factors influencing hatchability, etc., are easily accessible and will not be presented here. Full information may be found in Taylor (1949), Jull (1951), Landauer (1951), and Card (1952). The following remarks will be limited to a few essential details.

The most important prerequisite for successful operations is a supply of first-rate, strictly fresh eggs with a high percentage of fertility and a low percentage of abnormal development. The quality of the eggs should be tested rigorously before operations are started on a large scale. There is, apparently, no difference in quality between the different breeds.

Storage.—Eggs should not be stored longer than 6 days. They should be stored in a cool place. The optimal temperature for storage is around 50° F. (10° C.).

Incubators.—Two types are on the market: models without forced-air draft, in which the warm air diffuses downward onto the egg, and models with forced-air circulation. Smaller units are usually of the first type. They are entirely satisfactory for laboratory use but require more attention than the latter. Incubators are best installed in a room with even temperature and with good ventilation. They should not be exposed to direct sunlight. It is advisable to follow closely the directions of the manufacturer concerning temperature, humidity, etc.

Temperature.—In the still-air type, the temperature varies considerably in different levels of the incubator space. The temperatures 2–3 inches above the eggs (readings on hanging thermometers) are 1°–2° higher than temperatures on top of the eggs. The optimal temperature for incubators without forced-air draft is 102°–103° F. (38.9°–39° C.) throughout the incubation period (read-

143

ings on thermometers which are placed on top of the eggs). In forced-draft incubators the optimum is between 99° and 100° F. (37.2°–37.8° C.).

Humidity.—Humidity is an essential factor in successful incubation. Refilling of the water pans or of other devices for evaporation should be carefully attended to. In general, a relative humidity of 60 per cent was found to be optimal. The humidity in the incubator is, of course, closely related to the humidity in the room and to the ventilation within the incubator and in the room.

Turning the eggs twice daily seems to be essential for normal hatching. However, operated eggs with sealed windows should not be moved or disturbed.

Fertility, hatchability, mortality.—The natural breeding season is February to June, and the best material can be obtained during this season, but acceptable material can be obtained at almost any time except during hot summer months. Very cold weather reduces the percentage of fertility. Fertility and hatchability are not correlated with each other. A hatchability of 80 per cent, which implies an even higher percentage of fertility, is considered satisfactory. Two peaks of mortality occur during incubation, one around the second to fourth day and another around the nineteenth to twentieth day (see Landauer, 1951).

Testing by candling.—Candlers can be obtained from farm-supply houses, or they can be easily prepared in the following way: Make a circular hole approximately 2 inches in diameter in the bottom of a tin can. Mount a 100-watt bulb on a wooden base and invert the tin over it. Place the egg over the hole. Candle in a darkened room. The yolk-sac circulation becomes visible at $2\frac{1}{2}$–3 days of incubation as a network of blood vessels radiating from an indistinct dark spot, which is the embryo. In the following days the rocking movements of the embryo can be recognized in candling, and the expanding vitelline circulation, as well as the beginning chorio-allantoic circulation, can be seen. From the third to about the seventh day dead embryos can be recognized by the "blood ring"—blood settles at the periphery of the area vasculosa. From the seventh day on, the chorio-allantoic circulation can be seen in live embryos as an irregular network closely applied to the shell. From the thirteenth day on, living embryos appear increasingly dark, and the line of demarcation against the air chamber is very sharp and distinct. In embryos which die during these days this line is indistinct and hazy.

BIBLIOGRAPHY

CARD, L. E. 1952. Poultry production. 8th ed. Philadelphia: Lea & Febiger.
JULL, M. A. 1951. Poultry husbandry. 3d ed. New York: McGraw-Hill.
LANDAUER, W. 1951. The hatchability of chicken eggs as influenced by environment and heredity. Rev. ed. Storrs Agric. Exper. Sta. Bull. 262.
TAYLOR, L. W. 1949. Fertility and hatchability of chicken and turkey eggs. New York: Wiley.

2. STAGE SERIES

The stage series of Keibel and Abraham (1900) has been superseded by the stage series of Hamburger and Hamilton (1951; reprinted in Lillie-Hamilton, 1952), which is now rather universally adopted. It is based on readily identifiable structural characteristics rather than on chronology. All references to stages in the present manual refer to this series. The limb buds of 4 stages (17–20) that are widely used in experimental work are illustrated in Figure 31. These stages are characterized as follows:

Stage 17 (Fig. 31, a).—Wing and leg primordia are marked off as slight swellings. 29–32 somites. Incubation period: 52–64 hours.

Stage 18 (Fig. 31, b).—Wings are small buds; length: width = 5:1. 30–36 somites. Incubation period: 65–69 hours.

Stage 19 (Fig. 31, c).—Wings are median buds; length: width = 4:1. 37–40 somites. Incubation period: 68–72 hours.

Stage 20 (Fig. 31, d).—Wings are large buds; length:width = 3:1. 40–43 somites. Incubation period: 70–72 hours.

A corresponding series for the duck embryo has been worked out by Koecke (1958).

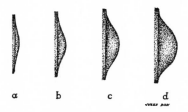

FIG. 31.—Some stages of wing buds of chick embryos. a = stage 17; b = stage 18; c = stage 19; d = stage 20 of the stage series of Hamburger-Hamilton (1951).

BIBLIOGRAPHY

HAMBURGER, V., and HAMILTON, H. 1951. A series of normal stages in the development of the chick embryo. Jour. Morphol., **88**:49.

KEIBEL, F., and ABRAHAM, K. 1900. Normentafel zur Entwicklungsgeschichte des Huhnes (*Gallus domesticus*). Jena: G. Fischer.

KOECKE, H. 1958. Normalstadien der Embryonal-Entwicklung bei der Hausente. Embryologia, **4**:55.

Lillie's Development of the chick. Rev. by HAMILTON, H. 1952. New York: Holt.

3. STANDARD EQUIPMENT FOR OPERATIONS ON CHICK EMBRYOS

Materials for joint use of the class

 incubator with turning trays and with hatching trays (wire trays). Lay out some of the turning trays with cotton strips on which the eggs are placed after the operation for further incubation. It is advisable to use 2 incu-

145

bators: one with turning trays for incubation before and after the operation (it should be opened as little as possible) and one with flat wire trays
on which the eggs in their "nests" are placed temporarily during the operation.

1 autoclave

1 candler

several "nests" on which eggs are placed during the operation. Place a pad-
ding of cotton on a watch glass. Mold a groove in the cotton in which the
egg will fit. "Nests" may also be made of foam rubber. From a pad, 1 inch
high, cut a piece, 2×3 inches, and carve out a groove in which the egg
fits. The nest can be glued on a piece of wood or plywood.

*paper towels[1]

*cotton, wrapped in paper towel and sealed with masking tape

*masking tape; to be sterilized every few days and used only when dry

*several large flasks with 0.9 per cent NaCl

agar plates, stained with neutral red and Nile blue sulfate, for vital staining
see p. 61)

Materials for each student

*5 watch glasses with lids

1 small scalpel

1 hack-saw blade

2 pairs of watchmaker forceps, carefully sharpened

1 iris knife

several fine lancets (sharpened sewing needles, p. 9)

needle-holder of wood

several fine glass needles

1 sharp steel needle to pierce hole in egg shell

1 pair fine scissors

1 pair large scissors

several wide-mouth pipettes

several small pipettes

1 micropipette

1 alcohol lamp

1 coplin jar with cotton on the bottom, filled with 70° alcohol, to keep fine
steel instruments clean

4. THE LUNDVALL TECHNIQUE OF CARTILAGE STAINING *in toto*
(After Lundvall, Anat. Anz., **25:** 1905; **27:** 1906)

Usually it is not feasible in courses of experimental embryology to section
the transplants. Therefore it is suggested that limb primordia be used for

[1] All items marked with an asterisk must be autoclaved.

chorio-allantoic, coelomic, and flank grafts. Cartilaginous limb skeletons of transplants, 9–13 days old, can be stained *in toto* within less than a week, using the simple method described below. For older, ossified skeletons the alizarin red method is recommended. It is suggested that normal (host) limbs be stained together with the transplants for comparison.

1. Fix in Bouin's fluid

> picric acid, sat. aq. sol. . . . . .75 parts
> 40 per cent formaldehyde. 25
> glacial acetic acid. 5

or in formaldehyde 1:10 for 1–2 days.

2. Wash in 70 per cent alcohol. After Bouin fixation add a few drops of lithium carbonate (saturated solution in 70 per cent alcohol). Change the fluid until the yellow color has completely disappeared.

3. Remove skin with feathers, adhering viscera, and fat masses. Use watchmaker forceps.

4. Stain in methylene blue (0.25 gm. per 100 cc. of 70 per cent alcohol, with 3 per cent of HCl, by volume), or in toluidin blue (same solution), for 2–3 days.

5. Destain in 70 per cent alcohol for at least 48 hours (change several times): in 95 per cent alcohol for 3–4 hours (change) and in absolute alcohol for 12 hours (change). In absolute alcohol the soft tissues should be completely destained, but the blue cartilage can be seen faintly through the other tissues.

6. Clear, harden, and store in 3 parts of oil of wintergreen plus 1 part benzyl benzoate.

B. EXPERIMENTS

The chick embryo lends itself to the same experimental procedures as the amphibian embryo: vital staining, extirpation, transplantation, and isolation of embryonic areas (see Rawles, 1952). A unique site for the isolation of parts is offered by the highly vascularized extra-embryonic membranes, particularly the chorio-allantoic membrane. All these in vivo techniques will be dealt with below. The tissue- and organ-culture methods have become highly specialized and are hardly adaptable to classroom experiments. Much use has been made of the so-called "watch-glass technique" of explantation of whole blastoderms of early stages, designed originally by Fell and Robison (1929) for organ culture. The blastoderm is removed from the yolk and transferred to the surface of a plasma or agar clot to which nutrient medium is added. The clot is prepared in a watch crystal that is placed in a moist chamber. Blastoderms can be reared for 1–3 days. The technique has been used for the study of morphogenetic movements by carbon-particle marking, for transection and similar experiments, and for the study of nutrient requirements. A simplified version of this technique for classroom use has been designed by Spratt (1947), and another useful modification by New (1955).

In the following we present first a general procedure for all in vivo experiments, and then detailed directions for a few selected experiments.

1. GENERAL PROCEDURE FOR OPERATIONS

It is necessary to use all precautions against contamination that are possible in an open laboratory, to sterilize all instruments, and to pull all steel instruments through the flame before they are brought in contact with the embryo. Expedite all operations to avoid long exposure of the embryo and cooling. At the beginning allow a sufficient number of eggs for each student, for practice. With a pencil mark on the blunt end the day and hour at which the incubation has begun. Remember that it takes some time for the egg to warm up and resume development. Determine the rate of development in your incubator and prepare a table correlating stages with hours of incubation. Have the stage series of Hamburger-Hamilton available for reference.

1. Prepare the *operation table*.—Spread the working space with sterile paper towels. Clean the microscope stage with cotton dipped in alcohol. Lay out glass instruments under a fold of paper towels and place steel instruments in jar with alcohol. Have burner, tape, and agar plates for vital staining ready.

2. *Candle* 3–4 eggs, in a dark corner of the laboratory. Locate the blastoderm. It is a darkish, circular area, which floats freely to the upper side. If necessary, shake or rotate the egg gently to facilitate the movement. The embryo can be recognized in the center at 2–2½ days if the shell is not too thick. Mark the center of the blastoderm or the location of the embryo with a circu-

148

lar or square pencil mark. Place the eggs on nests, marked side up; retain one for operation and return the others to the incubator.

3. *Prepare the window.*—Wipe the marked area and the blunt end with 70 per cent alcohol. With a sharp steel needle pierce the air space at the blunt end. The yolk will then settle, and the blastoderm will come to lie at some distance from the upper shell membrane, thus avoiding its injury when the shell membrane is removed. Using the hacksaw, gently, steadily, and without much pressure, saw through the shell on three sides of a rectangle $(1-1\frac{1}{2}$ cm.).[2] With some experience, it is possible to avoid injury to the shell membrane. Drop saline on the raw cuts and carefully loosen and raise the piece of shell with the forceps; break it off and discard it. The shell membrane is now exposed. If necessary, add saline to moisten it thoroughly. This precaution is taken to avoid injury to the blastoderm, in case it should still adhere to the inner surface of the shell membrane, and to facilitate the removal of the latter. Remove the membrane with the forceps and discard it. Avoid dropping of shell particles onto the blastoderm. Large particles should be removed with fine forceps (pull through flame) after moistening of the blastoderm. The embryo is now exposed.

4. Determine the stage and record it in your notebook or on the shell; proceed with the *operation*.

5. *Closing of window.*—With a clean pair of scissors, cut a piece of dry, sterile masking tape, considerably larger than the window. Center it over the opening and stick it onto the shell. The tape must adhere smoothly to the shell. Carefully flatten out all wrinkles with your thumbnail to avoid contamination. Do all these manipulations gently, with no great pressure; thin shells may crack.

6. Take a *record* of the operation, including stage of donor and host. Write the protocol number of the operation and your initials on the shell near the window and return the egg to the incubator. Gently place it on a tray, window facing upward. Disturb the operated eggs as little as possible. If you wish to check after a few days whether the embryo is alive, remove it gently from the incubator, very carefully peel off the tape from one side, and inspect the embryo under good illumination. Immediately seal the window again, using all precautions, as under section 5.

BIBLIOGRAPHY

FELL, H. B., and ROBISON, R. 1929. The growth, development and phosphatase activity of embryonic avian femora and limb buds cultivated in vitro. Biochem. Jour., **23**:767.

NEW, D. A. T. 1955. A new technique for the cultivation of the chick embryo. Jour. Embr. and Exper. Morph., **3**:326.

RAWLES, M. 1952. Transplantation of normal embryonic tissues. In The chick embryo in biological research. Annals N.Y. Acad. Sci., **55**:302.

SPRATT, N. T. 1947. A simple method for explanting and cultivating early chick embryos in vitro. Science, **106**:452.

[2] This can also be done with a dentist's drill.

2. PROSPECTIVE ORGAN-FORMING AREAS AND MORPHOGENETIC MOVEMENTS IN THE EARLY CHICK EMBRYO

INTRODUCTORY REMARKS

In the chick embryo, gastrulation proceeds in 2 phases: the formation of the hypoblast (endoderm) by delamination of cells from the upper layer (the epiblast), which is followed by the invagination of mesoderm through the *primitive streak*. The latter structure is of great importance in the early development of amniotes, not only as the site of mesoderm invagination, but also for the formation of the axial organs. The primitive streak originates at the posterior end of the area pellucida as a thickening of the epiblast (see Fig. 32). It lengthens in anterior direction until it extends to about $\frac{2}{3}-\frac{3}{4}$ of the length of the area pellucida. When it has reached its greatest extent ("definitive primitive streak," stage 4), it is a narrow ridge, terminating anteriorly in a round knob called "Hensen's node" (Fig. 34, *a*). A depression in the center of the node is called the "primitive pit." The primitive streak demarcates the main axis, and Hensen's node marks the head region of the future embryo. However, the anterior part of the head, including forebrain and eyes, is formed in front of Hensen's node.

From its inception, the primitive streak is not a stationary structure but is composed of continuously changing cell material. Lateral areas of the epiblast move toward the mid-line from both sides, then turn inside and spread again laterad between the epi- and the hypoblast, to form the mesodermal layer. The primitive streak is thus comparable to the blastopore of amphibians, except that invagination does not occur around free blastoporal lips but through a compact structure of densely packed cells. The primitive streak corresponds to the fused lateral lips, and Hensen's node to the dorsal lip, of an advanced amphibian gastrula.

Immediately after the definitive primitive-streak stage is reached, the formation of the embryo proper begins. The material for the embryo is supplied by the node and the streak and material adjacent to these structures, including also the underlying endoderm. The first visible sign of differentiation is the so-called "head process," an anterior extension of Hensen's node; it is composed of the anterior end of the notochord and the overlying medullary plate (Fig. 33). From this stage on, organ formation proceeds rapidly in anterior–posterior direction. Hensen's node regresses, and the primitive streak shortens, while the axial organs are built up in front of the node. The node always marks the boundary between the anterior organized part and the posterior part of the embryo, where gastrulation (mesoderm invagination) is still in progress. The elongation of the axial organs exceeds the shortening of the streak; as a result, the entire blastoderm lengthens and assumes a pear-shaped contour. Differentiation of the axial organs progresses in anterior–posterior sequence. While the neural tube is closing at the anterior end, the medullary plate is forming near the node; somite pairs segregate one after another.

The analysis of the morphogenetic movements during primitive-streak and embryo formation and the mapping of prospective organ-forming areas in the early blastoderm have met with considerable difficulties. The method of vital staining, which is not as reliable in the chick as in amphibian embryos, was supplemented by other methods, such as marking with carbon particles, chorio-allantoic grafts, and transection and excision experiments. The contributions of a number of investigators have been synthesized in the maps of Figure 32

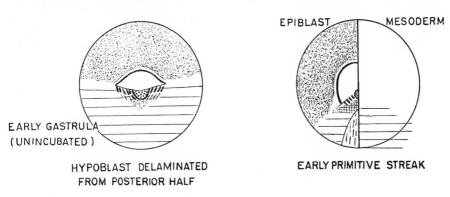

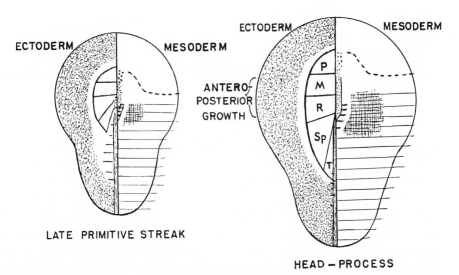

Fig. 32.—Maps of prospective organ-forming areas in four gastrulation stages of the chick embryo (from Rudnick, 1955, Fig. 113). In all but the first figure the left side shows areas located on the surface, and the right side invaginated mesoderm. Shaded areas = extraembryonic ectoderm. White areas = embryonic ectoderm. The medullary plate is inclosed in a heavy line. P = prosencephalon; M = mesencephalon; R = rhombencephalon; Sp = spinal cord; T = tail nerve cord. Stippled areas = notochord and prechordal plate. Heavy parallel lines = somites. Cross-hatching = heart. Light horizontal lines = lateral plate and extra-embryonic mesoderm. The dotted line in the lower figures indicates the anterior mesodermal border. Vertical shading = blastopore or primitive streak.

151

(from Rudnick, 1955; see also the reviews by Rudnick, 1944, 1948, and Waddington, 1952, and the papers of Spratt, 1947, 1952, 1955, 1957).

Special attention is called to the map of the definitive primitive-streak stage (Fig. 32, *lower left*), since this stage is used for our experiments. This map is best understood when related to those of earlier stages. The map of the un-incubated blastoderm (early gastrula) is comparable to the map of an early amphibian gastrula (Fig. 4); for instance, the main extent of the prospective axial organ areas is in both forms perpendicular to the main axis of the future embryo. During primitive-streak and embryo formation, we find the same basic morphogenetic movements; convergence, invagination, and elongation. All areas converge toward the median plane; as a striking example, the prospective medullary plate swings around to form a horseshoe-shaped field around the node and anterior streak. All mesoderm invaginates through the primitive

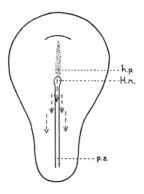

Fig. 33.—Head-process stage. The arrows indicate the movements of Hensen's node and adjacent material. *H.n.* = Hensen's node; *h.p.* = head process; *p.s.* = primitive streak (after Pasteels, 1937).

streak. The material which invaginates during the early phase of primitive-streak formation near the posterior end of the pellucid area spreads laterally and in posterior direction to form extra-embryonic mesoderm. Gradually, more anterior parts of the epiblast move inward and form the more anterior parts of the extra-embryonic mesoderm.

Of particular interest are localization and movements of the intra-embryonic mesoderm: notochord, somites, lateral plate. In the early gastrula this material has a position similar to that in amphibians, namely, posterior and adjacent to the prospective medullary plate. During the subsequent phases it invaginates at the level of the future Hensen's node and anterior primitive streak. At the definitive streak stage, invagination at the node level is completed but a small area of uninvaginated prospective mesoderm is still found in the epiblast adjacent to the anterior half of the primitive streak (see Fig. 32, *lower left*). The material which has invaginated at the node has been identified as prospective notochord and anterior somites. When the regression of the node starts, the anterior end of the notochord begins to differentiate in front of the node, forming the head process (Figs 32, 33). Its anterior tip will be found later at the border of forebrain and midbrain; it is continuous with the prechordal plate, which unlies the forebrain. The notochord elongates enormously as the node recedes and the primitive streak shortens. The elongation occurs mostly in the region immediately in front of the node. The node itself has always been recognized as the main source of notochord material, leaving prospective notochord cells in its wake while it recedes. However, refined marking experiments have shown that cells located behind the node also contribute to the notochord. Such cells lying in the path of the receding node are apparently picked up by the latter and subsequently incorporated in the notochord (Spratt, 1955, 1957).

We turn now to the localization and maps of the somites. At the definitive streak stage the anterior somite material has invaginated completely at the node level, where it occupies a position lateral to the notochord material (Fig. 32, *right side*). At this stage, the material for the more posterior somites is still outside, near the anterior streak (Fig. 32, *left side*), but it completes its invagination during the early phase of node regression and lines up adjacent to the notochord. Subsequently, it participates in the extensive elongation and backward shift of the axial organs. The same holds for the prospective spinal cord which up to the head-process stage is located near and somewhat posterior to the node, including the epiblast layer of the node itself. It should be realized that, while the flanking movements of the prospective medullary plate bring the two wings near the mid-line, no true concrescence, that is, no fusion of left and right halves in the mid-line, takes place. Rather, the median strip of the medullary plate (future floor of the neural tube) is formed by median epiblast, and the converging more lateral parts form the lateral walls and roof of the neural tube. The very extensive stretching of neural material (comparable to that in amphibians) can be demonstrated by vital-staining experiments.

According to this account, a deep vital-stain mark placed on the node and involving both epiblast and mesoderm would stain notochord, anterior somites, and the floor of the neural tube. A mark placed on the anterior part of the definitive primitive streak would stain posterior somites and lateral plate and occasionally the middle and posterior notochord. In order to stain the eye, the mark has to be placed in front of Hensen's node, slightly lateral to the median plane.

It should be understood that vital-staining experiments concern only the "prospective significance" of organ-forming areas (see p. 50). Their inherent potencies may be greater; they have been explored by chorio-allantoic grafts and excision and transplantation experiments.

BIBLIOGRAPHY

Rudnick, D. 1944. Early history and mechanics of the chick blastoderm. Quart. Rev. Biol., **19**:187.

————. 1948. Prospective areas and differentiation potencies in the chick blastoderm. Annals N.Y. Acad. Sci., **49**:761.

————. 1955. Teleosts and birds. In WILLIER, WEISS, and HAMBURGER (eds.), Analysis of development. Philadelphia: Saunders.

SPRATT, N. T. 1947. Regression and shortening of the primitive streak in the explanted chick blastoderm. Jour. Exper. Zool., **104**:69.

————. 1952. Localization of the prospective neural plate in the early chick blastoderm. *Ibid.*, **120**:109.

————. 1955. Analysis of the organizer center in the early chick embryo. I. Localization of prospective notochord and somite cells. *Ibid.*, **128**:121.

————. 1957. Analysis of the organizer center in the early chick embryo. II. Studies of the mechanics of notochord elongation and somite formation. *Ibid.*, **134**:577.

WADDINGTON, C. H. 1952. The epigenetics of birds. Cambridge, England: Cambridge University Press.

3. VITAL-STAINING EXPERIMENTS ON PRIMITIVE-STREAK STAGES

a) GENERAL PROCEDURE OF VITAL STAINING

In the chick embryo two methods have been used for the study of morphogenetic movements and for the mapping of prospective organ-forming areas in early blastoderm stages: vital staining and marking with carbon particles. The latter method, though more reliable than the former, does not lend itself readily to classroom experiments, for several reasons. It is not applicable to early blastoderms in vivo, because it would require the puncturing of the vitelline membrane, which results in abnormal development. For this reason, the extensive carbon-marking experiments of Spratt and others, which added greatly to our knowledge of morphogenetic movements and localization in early stages, were done on blastoderms explanted on a plasma or agar clot (p. 148). When applied to older stages, carbon particles placed under the ectoderm disappear and the embryo has to be cleared at the end of the experiment to make them visible. Students who wish to do carbon-marking experiments are referred to Spratt (1946) and Straus and Rawles (1953).

Following Vogt's experiments on amphibians, Wetzel (1929), Pasteels (1937), and others have used vital dyes (Nile blue sulfate and neutral red) for marking experiments. The results in the chick embryo are less satisfactory than those in amphibian embryos, because the dyes diffuse more readily and particularly neutral red fades out more rapidly than in amphibians. Furthermore, the dyed agar placed on the surface does not stain the epiblast selectively, but the dye diffuses into the hypoblast, and it is difficult to distinguish between the movements of the two layers. Other shortcomings of the method are discussed in Spratt (1947, Appendix C). Nevertheless, the method gives an impressive picture of some of the basic morphogenetic events in the early history of the chick embryo. The primitive-streak stage has been selected for the experiments described below to illustrate the movements leading to the formation of the head process, notochord, and other structures. Obviously, the same type of experiment can be done on other stages and other areas. Before

154

starting the experiments, the student should read section 2 (p. 150) and obtain a thorough understanding of the formation and fate of both the primitive streak and the embryo, in order to be able to interpret the experimental results. The illustrations in Wetzel and Pasteels (quoted above) will also be helpful in this respect.

Material for experiments 47–49

Embryos in the definitive primitive-streak stage (stage 4; incubation time approximately 16–20 hours), 6–8 eggs per student

standard equipment (p. 145)

for preparation of dyed agar plates see p. 61

Note.—Early embryos are very delicate; they have to be handled with utmost care. Furthermore, some samples of vital dyes, including Gruebler's Nile blue sulfate were found to be toxic to early chick embryos. Dyed agar should be tested before it is used in classroom experiments. It is advisable to inspect the vital-stained embryos as early as 6–8 hours after staining and then again 6–8 hours later. In this way some important observations can be made even if the embryo does not survive much longer. Neutral red is used for the "background" stain because it fades out more rapidly than Nile blue sulfate.

Procedure

Follow the general procedure, steps 1–4, page 148. It is not necessary to pierce the air space at the blunt end. After step 4, continue as follows:

5. Clean the dyed agar plates with cotton dipped in 70 per cent alcohol. Moisten small areas with sterile saline. After the agar is soaked, scrape off small pieces with a sterile knife or razor blade and place them in sterile saline. Allow clouds of excess dye to diffuse out. Cut out small pieces of appropriate size. The neutral red pieces should be large enough to cover the central part of the blastoderm; the blue pieces should be somewhat larger than Hensen's node and either square or narrow strips. Transfer these pieces to a dish with clean saline, using a micropipette.

6. The red agar piece is used to make the primitive streak visible. Place a square piece of red agar on the center of the blastoderm; transfer it either in a micropipette in a small drop of saline or with a pair of watchmaker forceps with very fine points. Carefully avoid an injury to the vitelline membrane. The dye diffuses instantly through the membrane. Check the staining process and remove the agar piece as soon as the faint contour of the primitive streak and of Hensen's node becomes visible. To avoid injury to the vitelline membrane, moisten the surface of the blastoderm before picking up the agar.

7. Transfer a small piece of blue agar to the embryo and place it in the desired position, using the point of a watchmaker forceps or a fine steel knife. Check the staining process and interrupt it when a distinct, but not too deep, mark is impressed on the embryo. Overstaining is dangerous. Staining takes

approximately 2–3 minutes, depending on the depth of impregnation and thickness of the agar piece.

8. Make a careful sketch of the precise location of the blue mark. This is absolutely necessary for the correct interpretation of the results.

9. Seal the window with masking tape; mark the protocol number and your initials on the shell and very gently return the egg to the incubator. It may be turned 90°, so as to place the embryo under the intact shell.

10. Make your first observations 6–8 hours after staining, and from then on every 6–8 hours. Use optimal illumination. Locate the blue mark and make careful sketches.

11. Terminate the experiment when development seems to be abnormal or, at any rate, not later than after 24 hours. Stain the whole embryo very lightly with neutral red and make a sketch; indicate the extent of the blue stain as accurately as possible. The embryos can then be dissected out by cutting the blastoderm at a safe distance from the embryo. Transfer the blastoderm in a wide-mouthed pipette to a dish with clean saline, remove adhering yolk, and locate the stained area under good illumination. Turn the blastoderm upside down. Make a sketch of the final position of the stain. Try to reconstruct the changes in the shape of the mark and its movements.

b) VITAL STAINING OF HENSEN'S NODE (FIG. 34, c–e)

EXPERIMENT 47

Procedure

Follow the directions given above. Place a piece of blue agar, somewhat larger than Hensen's node on the node. Avoid overstaining. After about 5 hours the "head-process stage" (stage 5) is reached. The head process and the receding node will be found stained. The blue line in front of the node is the anterior part of the notochord. Use strong illumination but avoid heating the embryo. Make observations and sketches every 6–8 hours and terminate the experiment after 24 hours. Cut out the blastoderm and locate the different structures and the extent of the stain. Turn the blastoderm upside down. Make a sketch.

c) VITAL STAINING AT THE ANTERIOR HALF OF THE PRIMITIVE STREAK (FIG. 34, *f*, *g*)

EXPERIMENT 48

Procedure

As before. Place a small piece of blue agar on the anterior part of the primitive streak, a short distance behind Hensen's node. Make intermittent observations and terminate the experiment after 24 hours. Follow directions for Experiment 47. The stain should include somites. Make a sketch.

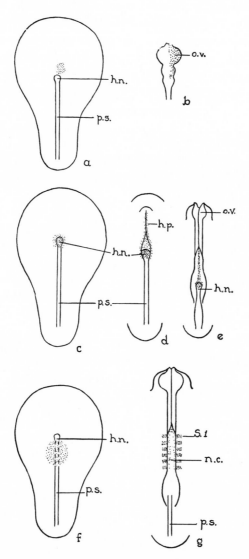

Fig. 34.—Vital-staining experiments in the primitive-streak stage (after Wetzel, 1929). *a, b* =
vital staining of a region in front of Hensen's node (prospective right forebrain and right eye). *a* =
immediately after staining; *b* = the same embryo, 24 hours later. *c–e* = vital staining of Hensen's
node: *c* = immediately after staining; *d* = 3 hours later; *e* = 24 hours later. *f, g* = vital staining
of the anterior part of the primitive steak: *f* = immediately after staining; *g* = 24 hours later. *h.n.* =
Hensen's node; *h.p.* = head process; *n.c.* = notochord; *o.v.* = optic vesicle; *p.s.* = primitive streak;
S1 = first somite.

d) VITAL STAINING OF THE PRENODAL AREA (FIG. 34, *a, b*)

EXPERIMENT 49

Procedure

As before. Place an oblong piece of blue agar immediately in front of Hensen's node. Make intermittent observations and terminate the experiment after 24 hours. Follow the directions for Experiment 47. Locate the stain in the forebrain and optic vesicles. Make a sketch.

BIBLIOGRAPHY

PASTEELS, J. 1937. Études sur la gastrulation des vertébrés méroblastiques. III. Oiseaux. Arch. de biol., **48**:382.

SPRATT, NELSON T., JR. 1946. Formation of the primitive streak in the explanted chick blastoderm marked with carbon particles. Jour. Exper. Zool., **103**:259–304.

———. 1947. Regression and shortening of the primitive streak in the explanted chick blastoderm. Jour. Exper. Zool., **104**:69–100.

STRAUS, W. L., JR., and RAWLES, M. E. 1953. An experimental study of the origin of the trunk musculature and ribs in the chick. Amer. Jour. Anat., **92**:471–510.

WETZEL, R. 1929. Untersuchungen am Hühnchen. Die Entwicklung des Keims während der ersten beiden Bruttage. Arch. f. Entw'mech., **119**:188.

4. CHORIO-ALLANTOIC GRAFTS

a) INTRODUCTORY REMARKS

Before starting these experiments, the student should review the formation and structure of the chorio-allantoic membrane in Lillie-Hamilton (see Fig. 35, *A*).

This isolation method makes use of the highly vascularized chorio-allantoic (C-A) membrane of avian embryos. It is sufficiently far developed in 8-day chick embryos to serve as a substrate for isolates, and it is easily accessible to the experimenter. B. H. Willier (since 1924) and his co-workers are largely responsible for the introduction of this method for the analysis of the early embryology of the chick. The structures whose potencies are to be tested are placed on the membrane through a window in the shell that is sealed up after the operation. The grafts become vascularized and can be reared for 9–10 days. Since the C-A membrane breaks down before hatching, the grafts have to be recovered on the eighteenth or nineteenth day of incubation (reviews in Rudnick, 1944; Rawles, 1952).

The transplants are completely isolated from the structures of the host embryo proper, so that inductive effects, etc., cannot obscure the results. On the other hand, the transplants, being incorporated in the blood circulation of the host, are exposed to hormones and other substances carried in the blood stream. In this respect the isolation is incomplete, and the possible effects of these agents on the differentiation of the transplant must be taken into consideration. Another limitation of the method lies in space limitation on the

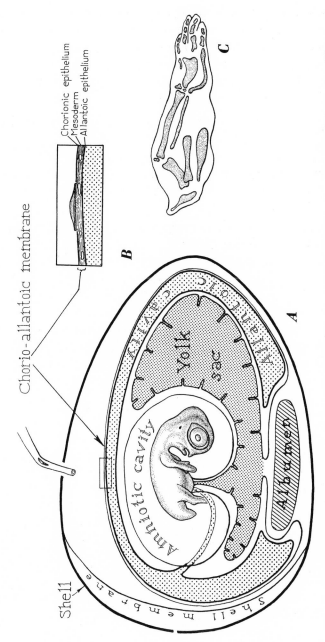

Fig. 35.—Chorio-allantoic grafting. $A = $ 10-day embryo. The air space at left has been punctured by a hole in the shell. The upper part of the chorio-allantoic membrane has dropped down. Transplant (limb bud) in micropipette introduced through window in shell. $B = $ detail of chorio-allantoic membrane. The chorionic epithelium has been lacerated at the site of implantation, and the limb bud oriented with its base facing downward. $C = $ a well-developed leg from a 3-day donor, grown for $10\frac{1}{2}$ days on the chorio-allantoic membrane (from Hunt, 1932).

membrane; transplants often flatten out and grow irregularly. In evaluating the results, one should be cautious not to attribute failures of normal development to the lack of inherent potencies of the transplanted primordia.

A promising new field was opened when it was found that mammalian tissue, including tumors, can be grown successfully on the C-A membrane. The membrane was also found to be a suitable substrate for the propagation of viruses and other micro-organisms (see Beveridge and Burnet, 1946). This enhances the usefulness of the C-A membrane for microbiological and medical research but also increases the danger of infection in grafting experiments.

b) CHORIO-ALLANTOIC GRAFTS OF LIMB PRIMORDIA

The experiment demonstrates that limb buds are capable of self-differentiation when isolated from the body at 2–3 days of incubation. This experiment was made first by Murray (1926; see 1936). This author grafted whole limb buds and proximal, distal, or longitudinal halves from 3- to 5-day embryos and found a rather rigid self-differentiation of fragments. For instance, the proximal part of a leg bud from a 3-day donor formed femur, and the distal part formed the tibiotarsus, the fibula, and the foot. However, experiments on the limb buds of 3-day chick embryos *in situ* showed that under appropriate conditions they are capable of regulation and duplication (Zwilling, 1956, and others). This should be a warning not to generalize in matters of determination from a limited set of data. In the explants the cartilages are often abnormal in shape and the skeletons incomplete because of unfavorable conditions on the membrane. Figure 35, *c*, shows an unusually well-differentiated graft (from Hunt, 1932).

EXPERIMENT 50

Material

10–12 eggs per student
standard equipment (p. 145)

Procedure

Read the general directions, p. 148.

INCUBATION

Start the incubation of hosts (5–6 eggs per student) 9–10 days before operation and the incubation of donors (same number per student) approximately 60–70 hours before operation, depending on the conditions in your incubator. The donor embryos should be in stages 18 or 19. Mark on each egg the date and hour at which incubation was started.

PREPARATION OF THE HOST EMBRYO

In the original technique a small window in the shell and shell membrane exposed the vascularized C-A membrane, which at 8–10 days of incubation is

160

closely applied to the shell membrane. The graft was then placed on the membrane and the window sealed. Under these conditions, the development of the graft located immediately under the shell was restricted by space limitations. Several investigators have overcome this difficulty by dropping the C-A membrane down onto the yolk sac and amnion before implantation of the graft, whereby unlimited space is provided for the expansion of the growing transplant. The same result can be achieved by settling the entire blastoderm at 2–3 days of incubation (see Zwilling, 1959). Both techniques are presented here. The latter avoids the hazard of injuring the C-A membrane when the window is opened.

1a. After the host eggs have been incubated for 2–3 days, they are candled and the position of the embryo is marked on the surface. The blunt end is pierced with a strong, pointed steel needle (pull through the flame), whereby the air escapes from the air chamber and the blastoderm settles down. At 9 days a small window is prepared in routine fashion (p. 149). Avoid sawing through the shell membrane and moisten the latter before removing it. This precaution is necessary because the blastoderm occasionally still sticks to the membrane; it will drop at the moment when the shell membrane is opened. The window is sealed with masking tape, and the egg is returned to the incubator, window facing upward. Place it on cotton.

1b. (*Alternative.*) After 9–10 days of incubation, when everything is prepared for the operation, candle the egg and mark a place, at some distance from the embryo, where a strong blood vessel bifurcates. Puncture the air chamber at the blunt end of the egg with a sharp steel needle. The release of air does not yet settle the C-A membrane; but it will drop as soon as the shell membrane is ruptured. This has to be done with great caution in order to avoid injury and hemorrhage in the closely adhering C-A membrane. Saw a very small window at the previously marked region. Drop saline on the raw cuts; carefully remove the piece of shell; flood the exposed shell membrane with saline and cautiously puncture the shell membrane with the forceps. One can observe the dropping of the C-A membrane at this moment. Enlarge the window somewhat until a well-vascularized area is exposed. Close the window with masking tape and return the egg to the incubator until the graft is prepared.

PREPARATION OF THE TRANSPLANT

2. Candle the donor embryo and mark its position. Place the egg on a cotton nest, pierce a hole in the blunt end with a strong, pointed steel needle, and saw a large square window at the marked region; avoid sawing through the shell membrane. Moisten the shell membrane over the embryo and remove it with the watchmaker forceps. The embryo is now exposed. Enlarge the window if necessary.

3. With a pair of fine scissors cut out the blastoderm a short distance from

the embryo. Transfer it to a watch glass containing sterilized saline, using the wide-mouthed pipette, or pick it up with a fine forceps. Determine and record the stage of the embryo. Discard the egg.

4. The embryo is covered with amnion and chorion. Rupture and remove these membranes very carefully with 2 watchmaker forceps or one forceps and a fine steel knife. Remove the pieces of blastoderm surrounding the embryo and discard them. Work under the low power of the binocular microscope against a dark background.

5. Locate the wing and the leg buds. Before isolating them, make two transverse cuts through the entire embryo, one through the neck and one between wing and leg buds (*x, y,* in Fig. 36, *a*). Use fine forceps for holding the embryo and a fine steel knife for the cutting. Next, dissect out one limb bud and adjacent somites. The somites provide for a broader base and thus facilitate spreading of the graft on the C-A membrane. Hold the piece with a forceps and dissect the limb bud with an iris knife or a steel needle with a very sharp edge. (Dip steel instruments in 70 per cent alcohol and pull them through the flame each time you use them.) The endoderm adhering to the inner surface may also be removed or trimmed. Cover the dish and put it aside.

TRANSPLANTATION

6. Take a host embryo out of the incubator; place it on a cotton nest and remove the tape over the window. The C-A membrane is now exposed. Notice the rocking movements of the embryo. For implantation choose a very well vascularized spot in the angle between bifurcating blood vessels, not too close to the embryo. Work under optimal illumination.

7. Suck the transplant into a Spemann micropipette and let it settle near its mouth. Under the binocular microscope drop it near the selected spot, with a very small amount of saline. The limb bud should face upward; if it lies upside down, add another drop of saline and turn it over. Remove all excess saline; the transplant should settle on the membrane and not float.

8. With the point of a very fine, sharp steel needle or iris knife very gently lacerate the surface layer of the C-A membrane without rupturing it. A slight hemorrhage is desirable; it seems to facilitate the incorporation of the graft. With the tip of a glass needle or steel knife move the transplant over the lacerated area.

9. Seal the window with masking tape. Record the protocol number and your initials on the shell and return the egg to the incubator without shaking or turning it. Place it on a tray laid out with cotton, window facing upward.

10. Immediately record all details of the operation, including stage of donor, age of host; record whether left or right bud, wing or leg, were grafted, how much somite material was retained, etc.

162

Note.—Repeat the experiment, using wing and leg buds. The same donor can supply several grafts.

11. During the following days check the transplants and record your findings. Vascularization should occur within a day. In opening, observe all safeguards against infection. Expose the window for as short a time as possible. Pull steel instruments through the flame.

RECOVERY OF THE GRAFT

Material

several finger bowls

several liters of warm saline (NaCl, 0.9 per cent, 38° C.)

a pair of strong scissors and a pair of fine scissors

watchmaker forceps

tissue lifter

Bouin's fixative (for Lundvall technique see p. 146) or alcohol-formalin (for modified van Wijhe technique see p. 196)

small vials with cork stoppers

labels

Procedure

The graft should be recovered when the host has reached an incubation age of 18–19 days.

12. Remove the tape and enlarge the window; avoid hemorrhage. Locate the transplant. Make a circular cut through the C-A membrane at a safe distance from the graft; the larger part of the graft may be below the surface. Cautiously lift the transplant out, on a tissue lifter or with a pair of forceps. Place it in a dish with saline, wash it, and trim the surrounding membrane. Inspect the graft closely, record your findings, and make a sketch if the transplant shows recognizable shape.

13. Drop the transplant in fixative; label the dish or vial with the protocol number and your initials. Discard the host embryo.

14. Follow directions for staining of cartilage and clearing (Lundvall technique, p. 146, or modified van Wijhe technique, p. 196). To your record add sketches of the stained skeleton and also sketches of the best cases obtained by others. Try to identify the skeletal elements.

c) CHORIO-ALLANTOIC GRAFTS OF EYE PRIMORDIA

The optic vesicle and optic cup are capable of development to advanced stages when isolated on the C-A membrane. If the graft "takes" well, it forms a large vesicle in which pigment epithelium, retina, iris, and lens are well differentiated.

EXPERIMENT 51

Material

Embryos between stages 12–16 (48–60 hours of incubation) are recommended as donors (4–5 eggs per student), but other stages may be used.

163

Hosts, 9–11 days (4–5 eggs per student)

standard equipment (p. 145)

Procedure

For preparation of host follow directions 1–4 in preceding experiment (p. 160).

5. *Preparation of transplant.*—Amputate the head by a transverse section at the hindbrain level. Hold the head with a forceps and cut out one eye and adjacent forebrain tissue to make the transplant more bulky. Avoid injury to the eye. Leave the epidermis, including lens epithelium, intact. For transplantation, follow directions 6–10 in the preceding experiment. Orient the transplant in such a way that the distal part of the eye faces upward.

Repeat the experiment several times. Both eyes of the donor may be used. Recover the graft on the eighteenth or nineteenth day; follow directions 12–13 in the preceding experiment. Fixation in 10 per cent formaldehyde. Clearing in Xylol or oil of wintergreen for permanent preservation. Clearing brings out the main structures; staining is not necessary.

d) CHORIO-ALLANTOIC GRAFTS OF SKIN

The main object of this experiment is the observation of feather differentiation. Study the appearance of feather germs and the growth of feathers in the Hamburger-Hamilton stage series and review feather development in Lillie-Hamilton. Study the feather tracts in 9- to 11-day embryos (stage 35–37).

EXPERIMENT 52

Material

donors, 5 to 6 days of incubation (stage 26–29; 4–5 per student)

hosts, 10–11 days (4–5 per student)

standard equipment (p. 145)

Procedure

For preparation of host follow directions 1–4 in Experiment 50 (p. 160).

5. Preparation of the transplant: Place the embryo in a caster or section dish of appropriate size. After removal of amnion and chorion, carefully strip off a piece of dorsal skin from the head region or between the wing or leg buds. Make a rectangular cut with a very sharp steel knife and strip the piece with a very fine forceps, holding the embryo with another forceps; or simply peel off a piece of skin with the forceps.

For transplantation follow directions 6–10 in Experiment 50 (p. 162). Orient the transplant in such a way that the dermis is spread on the C-A membrane. Recover the grafts at 18–19 days of incubation.

BIBLIOGRAPHY

BEVERIDGE, W. I. B., and BURNET, F. M. 1946. The cultivation of viruses and rickettsiae in the chick embryo. Med. Res. Council. Special Report Series, No. 256. London: H. M. Stationery Office.

HUNT, E. A. 1932. The differentiation of chick limb buds in chorio-allantoic grafts, with special reference to the muscles. Jour. Exper. Zool., **62:**57.

MURRAY, P. D. F. 1936. Bones. Cambridge, England: Cambridge University Press.

RAWLES, M. 1952. Transplantation of normal embryonic tissues in the chick embryo in biological research. Annals N.Y. Acad. Sci., **55:**302.

RUDNICK, D. 1944. Early history and mechanics of the chick blastoderm. Quart. Rev. Biol., **19:**187.

WILLIER, B. H. 1924. The endocrine glands and the development of the chick. I. The effects of thyroid grafts. Amer. Jour. Anat., **33:**67.

ZWILLING, E. 1956. Interaction between limb bud ectoderm and mesoderm in the chick embryo. II. Experimental limb duplication. Jour. Exper. Zool., **132:**173.

———. 1959. A modified chorio-allantoic grafting procedure. Transplantation Bull., **6:**115.

5. INTRA-EMBRYONIC TRANSPLANTATIONS

a) COELOMIC GRAFTS OF LIMB PRIMORDIA

The coelomic cavity of the chick embryo is an especially favorable site for the transplantation of primordia. It has certain advantages over the chorio-allantoic membrane: it allows for undisturbed expansion and normal morphogenesis of such primordia as limb buds and optic vesicles. Furthermore, it gives the transplant a longer life-span, since 3-day embryos are being used as hosts. The transplants are slipped through a hole in the somatopleure and attach themselves to the coelomic walls, mesenteries, or parts of the umbilical cord and receive blood supply from the host (Hamburger, 1938). Since transplants that develop at a distance from the central nervous system have little chance to receive a nerve supply, it is possible in this way to obtain non-innervated organs, for instance, completely nerveless limbs. They were found to be remarkably normal, particularly with respect to their skeletons and their joints (Hamburger, 1939; Hamburger and Waugh, 1940). Non-innervated musculature will undergo normal differentiation and cross-striation; but innervation is required for its maintenance, and, in its absence, the muscles degenerate shortly after their initial differentiation. These cases demonstrate that innervation and functional activity during development play only a minor role as causal factors in limb morphogenesis. Other primordia have been reared successfully in the coelomic cavity, as for instance, optic vesicles, spinal cord, and mouse tissue, including mouse tumors.

EXPERIMENT 53

Material

3–4 donors and 3–4 hosts per student
standard equipment (p. 145)
agar stained with neutral red

165

Procedure

Start the incubation of both donors and hosts about $2\frac{1}{2}$–3 days before the operation. They should be in stages 18 or 19 when operated on.

Cut out small pieces of red agar for vital staining and place them in sterile saline solution. Their size can best be determined when the first embryo is stained. It should be large enough to cover the right half of the embryo posterior to the tenth somite. Prepare half a dozen agar pieces. They must be replaced by fresh pieces when they begin to fade. Make other preparations as in sections 1–4 on page 148.

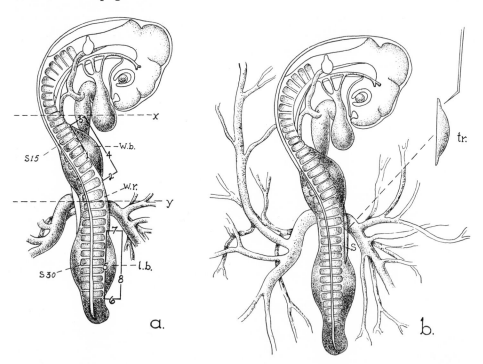

Fig. 36.—Limb-bud transplantation in the chick embryo. a = donor embryo; b = host embryo (both 34 somites, 72 hours of incubation). $l.b.$ = leg bud; s = slit for the reception of the transplant; $S15, S30$ = somites 15, 30; $tr.$ = transplant; $w.b.$ = wing bud; $w.r.$ = Wolffian ridge; for other letters and numbers see text.

VITAL STAINING OF THE HOST EMBRYO

5. Candle the egg. If the embryo is stuck on the side, it is often possible to bring it into the desired position on top by gentle shaking or rolling. With pencil, mark a square of about $1\frac{1}{2}$ sq. cm. on the shell above the embryo.

6. Place the egg on a nest, marked side up; pierce the blunt end with a steel needle, swab the surface with 70 per cent alcohol, and saw a square window as marked. Very carefully avoid sawing through the shell membrane and thus injuring the embryo. Hemorrhages are usually fatal. Saw slowly and steadily.

166

Saw only three sides and break the fourth side when the window is lifted up with the scalpel. Avoid the loosening of small shell particles on the edges of the window.

7. Moisten the shell membrane thoroughly with saline to avoid hemorrhages. Under the binocular dissecting microscope remove it very cautiously in the area of the window, using a pair of watchmaker forceps. The embryo should now be exposed. If it sticks on one side, roll or shake the egg gently and try to move it to the top. Add sufficient sterile salt solution to keep it moist. The embryo should settle rather deeply under the shell.

8. For vital staining place a piece of red agar over the right flank, covering the right wing bud and the region posterior to it. Cover the window with masking tape. Mark the egg with your initials and with a serial number and return it to the incubator for 5–10 minutes.

Note.—If the agar piece is deep red and rather thick, then it is best to stain through the vitelline membrane. The latter stains first but will soon give off all dye to the adjacent tissues. Otherwise, rupture the vitelline membrane with the watchmaker forceps before staining, then place the agar directly on the embryo and thus obtain a deep stain within a short time. Avoid overstaining.

PREPARATION OF THE TRANSPLANT

9. Candle another egg, marking the embryo as before. Place the egg on a nest and break or saw a large hole, considerably wider than that in the host, so that the embryo and the adjacent area vasculosa are laid open. With a pair of (sterilized) scissors cut out the entire area vasculosa with the embryo in its center. With the watchmaker forceps or with a wide-mouthed pipette transfer it to a dish with salt solution.

10. Under the binocular microscope turn the blastoderm right side up, flatten it, and hold it with the left forceps. Use a dark background. Locate wing and leg buds. Count the somites, determine the stage, and record these data. Amputate the head with an iris knife or sharp steel lancet (level x in Fig. 36, a) and discard it. Hold the embryo with the left forceps and cut out the right wing or leg bud with the iris knife. Make four cuts: the first, longitudinal and median to the bud, close to the somites; the second and third, perpendicular to this, in front of and behind the bud; and the fourth, lateral and not too close to the bud (*1, 2, 3, 4,* or *5, 6, 7, 8* in Fig. 36, a). The endoderm may be peeled off, using 2 forceps; but this is a rather delicate procedure and is not necessary. When the transplant is isolated, cover the dish with a lid and put it aside.

PREPARATION OF THE SITE OF IMPLANTATION IN THE HOST EMBRYO

11. Reopen the host embryo, add saline, and under the binocular microscope remove the agar with a pair of watchmaker forceps. Shake the embryo gently if the blastoderm adheres to the edge of the window.

167

12. If the amnion and chorion cover the operation region, it is necessary to slit them open. This is done with a glass needle. Hold the egg shell with your left hand; insert the needle into the amniotic cavity in the mid-line, where the raphe (suture) is visible, and with a jerky upward movement of the needle rupture the membranes. Continue this until at least the posterior half of the right wing bud is exposed. The membranes require no further care. They will heal back over the embryo.

13. The transplant is to be implanted through a hole posterior to the wing bud (*s* in Fig. 36, *b*). Locate wing and leg buds and vitelline arteries. In the following steps it is absolutely necessary to avoid hemorrhages. Be sure not to get too close to the lateral edges of the somites to avoid puncturing of the posterior cardinal vein, which runs underneath the lateral edges of the somites. Do not push the needle too deeply, to avoid injury to the splanchnic layer, which is highly vascularized. Under the binocular microscope (high power) push the glass needle through the somatopleure at a point between the wing and the leg bud and a short distance lateral to the outer edges of the somites, which stand out clearly in red. From this hole work forward and backward and make a longitudinal slit in the somatopleure parallel to the main axis and just large enough to allow the limb bud to slip through. Add saline to keep the embryo moist.

TRANSPLANTATION

14. Under the binocular microscope suck the prepared limb bud into the distal part of a micropipette. By gentle pressure on the rubber membrane which covers the lateral hole, drop the transplant onto the host near the slit. This should be done under the binocular microscope (low power) to avoid the loss of the transplant. Hold the egg shell with your left hand and manipulate the transplant through the slit into the coelom, using the tip of the glass needle (Fig. 36, *b*). The transplant may be oriented during or after the implantation. If one wishes to have the transplant adhere to the umbilical cord, it has to be pushed into a lateral position, at a considerable distance from the somites. Otherwise, leave it near the somites above the root of the vitelline artery in longitudinal orientation. Add a small amount of saline. Take a record; note whether wing or leg has been transplanted; note orientation, stage of host, etc.

15. Seal the window with a piece of masking tape. Return the egg to the incubator. Place it on a strip of cotton, the window facing upward.

RECOVERY OF THE TRANSPLANT

16. Allow the host to develop for 7–9 days; the best stage for fixation is 10–12 days of incubation, but good limb development can be observed in 8-day embryos, that is, 5–5½ days after operation. Do not roll the eggs during

this period. Prepare a pan or finger bowl with warm saline. Remove the window and widen the hole. Carefully dissect away the chorio-allantoic membrane. Carefully sever the umbilical cord and lift the embryo into the dish of saline. If no transplant is visible from the outside, it may be entirely hidden inside the coelomic cavity or it may have been resorbed. Carefully slit open the ventral body wall slightly to the left (apparent right) of the median line and inspect the inside of the body cavity. Fix the host embryo, together with the transplant, in Bouin and stain them with methylene blue (p. 146) to make the host and the transplant skeleton visible. Take careful records.

Dossel (1954) has described a method of intracoelomic grafting that makes use of older embryos of $3\frac{1}{2}$–4 days of incubation (stages 20–22) and permits the implantation of larger pieces of tissue. An opening is made in the chorion outside the embryo, and the implant is pushed past the allantois into the intra-embryonic coelom, where it can be lodged in any desired location. It is suggested that this method be tried, using limb or other primordia as implants.

b) FLANK GRAFTS OF LIMB PRIMORDIA

The method of implantation into the coelomic cavity has the disadvantage that the transplants cannot be fixed in a desired position. If a definite orientation is desired, the primordia are best implanted in the outer body wall. Flank grafts also permit the study of nerve ingrowth. The following experiment is based on Hamburger (1938, 1939).

EXPERIMENT 54

Material

> 2–3 donors and 3–4 hosts per student
> standard equipment (p. 145)

Procedure

As in Experiment 53, with the following modifications:

10 (p. 167). Preparation of the transplant. In cutting out the limb bud, leave small strips of tissue (somites or adjacent mesoderm) attached to the anterior and posterior ends of the base of the bud; these will be tucked into the slit. The other limb buds may be used for further transplantations.

13 (p. 168). Preparation of the slit in the host embryo. Make the slit between wing and leg bud as close to the somites as possible and not too long. Rather, lengthen it while you implant.

14 (p. 168). Implantation. With the tip of the glass needle tuck first the anterior end and then the posterior end of the limb bud into the slit (see Fig. 36, *b*). If the hole is slightly shorter than the bud, the transplant will be held in position by the tension of the tissues. The major part of the transplant should be exposed and its base closely applied to the somites of the host. No

other precaution is necessary to keep the transplant in position. If the transplant slips into the coelom, it can be recovered with the tip of the glass needle.

15 (p. 168). In handling the egg after the operation, be exceedingly cautious; avoid all sudden or jerky movements. Place it on cotton in the incubator and do not disturb it for a day or two.

c) FLANK GRAFTS OF EYE PRIMORDIA

The first flank grafts of optic vesicles were made by Alexander (1937) in connection with the problem of lens induction. Gayer (1942) obtained well-formed eyes by the same method, using optic vesicles of 10- to 20-somite stages. The shape and structures of the transplants were normal. This demonstrates the high degree of self-differentiating capacity of the optic vesicle with respect to its surrounding structures. However, practically all flank grafts showed a deficiency in the closure of the choroid fissure, of the type which is occasionally found as a congenital abnormality in human eyes, known in ophthalmology as "coloboma."

EXPERIMENT 55

Material
>   2–3 donors, stages 11–14; 3–4 hosts, stages 16–18, per student
>   standard equipment (p. 145)

Procedure

As in Experiment 53, with the following modifications:

Start the incubation of the host embryos 2–2½ days, and the incubation of the donors 36–48 hours, before operation. Exact incubation time depends on the temperature conditions of your incubator.

8 (p. 167). Vital stain the right-wing level rather than more posterior parts of the host.

10 (p. 167). Cut out the right optic vesicle, together with the right half of the forebrain. First, make a transverse cut behind the right optic vesicle through the head to the mid-line. Second, make a median cut through the anterior part of the head. The left eye may be used for another transplantation (Fig. 37, *b*).

13 (p. 168). Make the slit at the base of the wing, at about the level of the twentieth somite (Fig. 37, *a*).

14 (p. 168). Transfer the optic vesicle with adhering brain tissue onto the host blastoderm, using the micropipette. Drop it near the slit. With the tip of the glass needle tuck the brain portion into the slit, thus leaving the optic vesicle exposed on the surface (Fig. 37, *d*).

16 (p. 168). Incubate the host for not more than 9–10½ days (total age), i.e., 7–8 days after operation, at which stage all essential eye structures are

differentiated. In order to make visible such details as lens, retina, iris, choroid fissure, etc., without sectioning the transplant, the embryo may be fixed in Bouin, dehydrated, and cleared in oil of wintergreen.

d) TRANSPLANTATION OF NEURAL CREST FROM DARK TO WHITE BREEDS
TO DEMONSTRATE THE ORIGIN AND MIGRATION
OF MELANOPHORES

The dark pigment of vertebrates is contained in granular form in pigment cells, the so-called "melanophores." They originate in all vertebrates in the

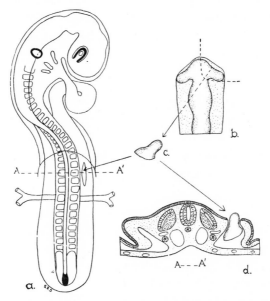

FIG. 37.—Transplantation of an optic vesicle in the chick (after Gayer, 1942). *a* = host embryo (30 somites, 60 hours of incubation) with slit for the implantation of the optic vesicle; *b* = head of the donor embryo (12 somites, 36 hours of incubation); the dotted lines indicate the cuts by which the right optic vesicle and the adjacent brain part are severed; *c* = transplant; *d* = cross-section through *a*, in level *A–A'*, showing the transplant in position.

neural crest; this has been demonstrated by extirpation, transplantation, and in vitro experiments (see reviews by DuShane, 1944; Rawles, 1948, 1955). Like all other neural crest cells, the embryonic melanophores, or melanoblasts, are wandering cells. They migrate from the dorsal part of the neural tube to their final locations, where they proliferate and form complex pigment patterns. In birds, they migrate into the developing feather germs and deposit pigment granules in the barb primordia. The remarkable migratory and pattern-forming capacities of melanophores were demonstrated in a classical experiment designed by Willier and Rawles (1938, 1940). A small piece of embryonic head epidermis from a dark breed of fowl, including some prospective

171

melanophores, was transplanted to the base of the wing bud of a 2–3-day embryo of a white breed. The transplanted epidermis was not incorporated in the epidermis of the host, but the melanoblasts adhering to it migrated into host territory. They settled down in the developing feather germs of the host wing and deposited their pigment. As a result, the fully developed wing was partly or entirely covered with black down feathers, all other feathers being uncolored. In some cases the pigmented area extended as far as to the ventral mid-line of the body. The melanophores thus exhibited not only an extensive migration but an extraordinary proliferative capacity; they all originated from the few neural-crest cells that adhered to the epidermal transplant.

Willier and Rawles and their associates carried the experiment further. The hosts were allowed to hatch. In due time the down feathers were replaced by the adult plumage. White Leghorn wings that carried a transplant of Barred Rock melanophores exhibited a typical barring pattern in their feathers. These and many similar experiments demonstrate clearly that the color pattern is largely determined by the genetic constitution of the melanophores rather than by that of the feathers themselves. However, the host-feather germs modify and control the activity of the melanophores to a certain extent. The role of both partners in the determination of the final pattern was analyzed by means of extensive series of reciprocal transplantations between many different breeds of fowl (reviews in Willier, 1948; Rawles, 1948, 1955).

EXPERIMENT 56

Material

> donors: any dark breed, e.g., Brown Leghorns, 3–4 eggs per student
> hosts: 4–5 eggs, White Leghorn; should be stage 17 or 18 but not older;
> > donors of the same stage or younger
> standard equipment (p. 145)

Procedure

Start the incubation of the donors and hosts 2½–3 days before operation. Proceed as in 1–4 (p. 148) and 5–7 (p. 166).

8. Prepare the slit in the host: Rupture chorion and amnion over the right wing bud. Open up a large hole. The membranes will heal over again. With the glass needle make a small but rather deep cut at the base of the wing and enlarge it to a small hole. Vital staining is not necessary. Return the host to the incubator.

9. Vital stain the head skin on the donor. Place a piece of red agar on the head in front of the otocyst. Stain for 5–10 minutes.

10. Meanwhile take the host out of the incubator; place it within easy reach. When the skin of the donor is sufficiently stained, cut out the transplant as follows: With the glass needle or watchmaker forceps strip a piece of skin

172

from the dorsal and dorsolateral surface of the head, in front of the otocysts. This piece contains neural-crest cells.

11. Transfer this piece directly onto the host, using the micropipette.

12. Implant the graft in the prepared slit; bury it deeply. Be sure that the transplant sticks to the slit.

13. Seal the window with masking tape and return the egg to the incubator, the window facing upward. Mark the egg with your initials and a protocol number.

14. Recover the host about 2 weeks after the operation. Pigment has formed at that stage and the down feathers have developed. Study the color of the wing, the extent of the pigmented area, etc. (see papers quoted above).

BIBLIOGRAPHY

ALEXANDER, L. E. 1937. An experimental study of the role of optic cup and overlying ectoderm in lens formation in the chick embryo. Jour. Exper. Zool., **75**:41.

DOSSEL, W. E. 1954. New method of intracoelomic grafting. Science, **120**:262.

DuSHANE, G. P. 1944. The embryology of vertebrate pigment cells. II. Birds. Quart. Rev. Biol., **19**:98.

GAYER, H. K. 1942. A study of coloboma and other abnormalities in transplants of eye primordia from normal and Creeper chick embryos. Jour. Exper. Zool., **89**:103.

HAMBURGER, V. 1938. Morphogenetic and axial self-differentiation of transplanted limb primordia of 2-day chick embryos. Jour. Exper. Zool., **77**:379.

———. 1939. The development and innervation of transplanted limb primordia of chick embryos. *Ibid.*, **90**:347.

——— and WAUGH, M. 1940. The primary development of the skeleton in nerveless and poorly innervated limb transplants of chick embryos. Physiol. Zoöl., **13**:367.

RAWLES, M. E. 1948. Origin of melanophores and their role in development of color patterns in vertebrates. Physiol. Rev., **28**:383.

———. 1955. Skin and its derivatives. In WILLIER, WEISS, and HAMBURGER (eds.), Analysis of development. Philadelphia: Saunders.

WILLIER, B. H. 1948. Hormonal regulation of feather pigmentation in the fowl. Special Pub. N.Y. Acad. Sci., **4**:321.

——— and RAWLES, M. E. 1938. Feather characterization as studied in host-graft combinations between chick embryos of different breeds. Proc. Nat. Acad. Sci., **24**:446.

———. 1940. The control of feather color pattern by melanophores grafted from one embryo to another of a different breed of fowl. Physiol. Zoöl., **13**:177.

PART IV
REGENERATION

A. GENERAL REMARKS

The remarkable phenomenon of regeneration demonstrates that the capacity for growth and differentiation is not limited to embryonic stages but persists throughout the life span of an organism. The regenerative potencies vary greatly among animals. Some protozoans, hydra and other coelenterates, the planarians among the Platyhelminthes, and the urodeles among the vertebrates are known for their extraordinary regenerative power. In higher animals, regeneration is restricted to tissue repair and renewal, such as wound-healing, nerve-fiber regeneration, continuous replacement of red blood cells and of keratinized epidermis cells, etc. For an extensive survey of the regenerative potencies of different groups see Korschelt (1927), and for brief surveys see Needham (1952), Nicholas (1955), and Hamburger (1960).

It has long been recognized that the repair of lost parts can be accomplished in two ways: by internal reorganization and transformation of old tissues without addition of new growth or by outgrowth of new tissue from the cut surface in the form of a regeneration bud or "blastema." Head and tail regeneration in *Planaria*, limb and tail regeneration in *Urodela*, are examples of the latter type. The change in shape, as well as the formation of a new pharynx by the old tissue in the regeneration of *Planaria*, is an example of the former type. In many instances both types are combined in the same form, and there may be no fundamental difference between them; but for practical purposes it is desirable to designate them by different technical terms. Morgan (1901) distinguishes between "epimorphosis" (proliferation of new tissue) and "morphallaxis" (changes within the old tissue) and includes both under the general heading "regeneration." Child (1941, p. 30) uses the term "reconstitution" to include all types and defines "regeneration" in the narrower sense as reconstitution by outgrowth and "reorganization" as reconstitution by internal changes.

In the majority of cases, precisely those parts that were removed are regenerated. However, there are instances in which more, or less, than was lost is regenerated, and there are cases in which the regenerated structure is different from the lost part (heteromorphosis). We shall give some examples of such instances below.

The regeneration processes are in many ways comparable to embryonic processes, and they pose the same problems of progressive differentiation and determination as have been dealt with in preceding chapters. In addition, there are problems which are peculiar to regeneration. For instance, there is the question of the initiation of regeneration, which is not always a matter of cre-

177

ating a wound surface; the case of lens regeneration in urodeles illustrates this point (see p. 197). There is the much discussed question of the origin of the regeneration material, which will be discussed briefly below. The determination problem itself assumes a new dimension: If a salamander limb is amputated at different levels, a different set of organizing factors is required at each level, to account for the fact that in each instance the regenerate is different, and always complementary to the stump. Similar questions arise when a whole hydra or planaria or a starfish regenerates from an arbitrarily chosen fragment. The notion of "morphogenetic fields" (p. 100) is applicable here, and the concept of "regeneration fields" has been developed by Weiss, Guyenot, and others, particularly with reference to regeneration in urodeles (see Weiss, 1939; Waddington, 1956). The young regeneration blastema with its underlying stump has several of the characteristics of a morphogenetic field discussed on p. 101. In its early stages the blastema has regulative properties, as is borne out by its capacity to form duplications—in other words, it passes through a stage in which it is determined as a whole but does not represent a mosaic of parts. Regeneration fields, like embryonic fields, extend beyond the boundaries of the organs which they represent: If a urodelan limb is extirpated, tissue adjacent to it will regenerate a complete limb. Regeneration fields, like embryonic fields, do have definite limits, however, and regeneration no longer occurs if a large area at the base of the limb or tail is removed. In this sense, regeneration is under the control not of the organism as a whole but of local agencies residing in the regeneration field. We know very little of these organizing factors and of the interactions between the stump and the blastema that result in the organization of the regenerate; and it should be understood that the term "regeneration field" has no explanatory meaning. Nevertheless, it is a very useful term, because it sums up, and focuses on, a complex and recurrent phenomenon that is basic to embryogenesis and regeneration.

The *gradient theory* of C. M. Child deserves a brief comment because it has been widely applied by Child and others to interpret regeneration phenomena, particularly the retention of the original polarity in regenerating fragments. The gradient theory is an ingenious attempt to unify developmental, restitutive, and reproduction processes in a single frame of reference. According to the theory, all structural differentiations in the early embryo, in regenerates and in asexual reproduction in invertebrates and plants, are preceded by quantitative differences in physiological activities that follow a definite gradient pattern. The apical end of a growing blastema or bud, the anterior end of a fragment of a planaria or hydra, or the animal pole of an egg usually shows the highest metabolic activity, and the decrement of activity usually follows the main axis (hence "axial gradients"). The fate of a group of developing or regenerating cells is determined primarily by its relative position in the gradient system: In a transversely cut piece of a planaria or hydra, the anterior

178

cut surface determines head formation because it has the relatively highest level of physiological activity in the system, the tail develops at the lowest level, and intermediate structures, such as the pharynx, are related to intermediate levels of activity. Polarity is thus conceived as a dynamic property of the whole system. When a fragment is isolated, it retains its inherent gradation of physiological activities and, with it, its polarization. In this connection, the experimental reversal of polarity (polar heteromorphosis) is of particular interest. One such instance, in short posterior pieces of planarians, will be discussed below (p. 185). The idea of "physiological dominance" is an integral part of Child's theory. The blastema forming at the region of highest activity (the head-forming blastema in the case of planarian regeneration) sets itself up as a "dominant region." It organizes the more caudal parts, including reorganization in the old piece and, at the same time, suppresses the formation of another head-forming blastema anywhere else. In this way the individuality in the regenerate is guaranteed. Duplications can occur if two separate dominant regions are produced experimentally in an individual. If the anterior part of a planaria is first transected and then split in the mid-line (Fig. 39, c, d), then two separate anterior cut surfaces are created, and an anterior duplication results. We cannot consider the many other facets of the theory or the extensive work that has been done by Child and his school to demonstrate the existence of gradients in a great variety of forms, with a variety of methods. We refer to his latest book (1941), which contains also an extensive bibliography.

It will become evident in the experiments discussed below that regeneration phenomena require a dynamic approach and that they strongly suggest an epigenetic concept of development. It is the merit of the gradient theory to emphasize this viewpoint. Gradient systems undoubtedly have to be given serious consideration, in the analysis of development and regeneration, as integrative and, in some instances, determinative mechanisms, though not to the exclusion of other mechanisms, as Child is inclined to believe. On the other hand, what has been said above of the "field" concept holds equally for the axial gradient theory: While its value as a unifying concept is uncontested, it has little explanatory value, because the physiological activities on which it is based have not been identified so far.

We have limited the experimental part on regeneration to 2 groups, the planarians and the urodeles, both of which are easily available. Additional experiments on protozoans, hydra, and fresh-water oligochaetes can be designed by the instructor wherever such material can be obtained.

BIBLIOGRAPHY

(See also p. xvii)

CHILD, C. M. 1941. Patterns and problems of development. Chicago: University of Chicago Press.

HAMBURGER, V. 1960. Regeneration (revised), in Encyclopaedia Britannica.

KORSCHELT, E. 1927. Regeneration und Transplantation. Vol. 1. Berlin: Borntraeger.

MORGAN, T. H. 1901. Regeneration. New York: Macmillan.

NEEDHAM, A. E. 1952. Regeneration and wound-healing. London: Methuen.

NICHOLAS, J. S. 1955. Regeneration, vertebrates. In WILLIER, WEISS, and HAMBURGER (eds.), Analysis of development. Philadelphia: Saunders.

WADDINGTON, C. H. 1956. Principles of embryology. New York: Macmillan.

WEISS, P. 1939. Principles of development. New York: Holt.

B. REGENERATION IN PLANARIA

1. LIVING MATERIAL: CULTURE METHODS

Two native species are commonly used for experiments: *Dugesia tigrina* Girard (= *Planaria maculata*) and *D. dorotocephala* Girard (= *Pl. dorotocephala*). They can be distinguished readily as follows:

Dugesia dorotocephala is larger than *tigrina* (length up to 25 mm.); it is uniformly dark (brown or black); its auricles are elongated and pointed (Fig. 38, *a*); it lives in springs and spring-fed streams and can be collected by baiting. It is found in middle-western states.

Dugesia tigrina is, at best, 15–18 mm. long; it is variable in color; usually it shows a spotted color pattern (white, irregular spots on a brownish or blackish background) or a light mid-dorsal stripe. Its auricles are broader and blunter than those of *D. dorotocephala* (Fig. 38, *b*). It lives in ponds, lakes, and slow-flowing streams on the under surface of stones and leaves and can be

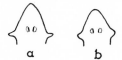

a   b

Fig. 38.—*a* = head of *Dugesia* (*Planaria*) *dorotocephala; b* = head of *D. tigrina* (*Pl. maculata*) (from Hyman, 1931).

collected by turning these over. Its distribution is eastern and middle-western states, west to the Mississippi, south to the Carolinas.

Culture of planarians.—Planarians collected in the field or bought from a dealer may be kept in large glass containers or dark enamel dishpans. They should be covered and kept in a dark, cool place. They are negatively phototactic and sensitive to light. They should be protected from strong illumination. Spring or well water is preferable to tap water. Planarians should be fed twice a week with strips of calf or beef liver. Before feeding, lower the water to a depth of a few inches. Distribute the strips of meat and remove them after 2–3 hours of feeding. Thereafter rinse the dish or pan thoroughly and fill it with fresh water. The animals are very sensitive to fouling of water. (For more details see Hyman, 1937.)

2. GENERAL EXPERIMENTAL PROCEDURE

Since the eighteenth century, *Planaria* has been one of the favorite materials for the study of regeneration. The voluminous literature on the subject is reviewed in Korschelt (1927), Child (1941, and previous books), and Brondsted (1955). A large number of cutting experiments can be done as class ex-

181

periments. In the following only a few experiments were selected. Others may be taken from the literature.

Material for Experiments 57–66

    Dugesia dorotocephala or *D. tigrina,* about 12 specimens per student and per experiment (Species differences exist with respect to regenerative power, time of regeneration, etc. Since the speed of regeneration varies with temperature, it is desirable to run all experiments at constant temperatures.)

    finger bowls or Petri dishes or paraffined paper cups

    pipettes

    small brush to transfer planarians

    The cutting is best done with a piece of razor blade on a cork disk. Break a double-edged razor blade in two, and break off pieces large enough to be held between your fingers. They may also be glued to a glass handle. Slice a cork about 1 inch in diameter into disks ½ inch or less in thickness.

General procedure for Experiments 57–66

    Note.—Use only pond or spring water. Do not feed experimental animals for a week before operations or while they regenerate. For each experiment select 8–10 specimens of as uniform size as possible. Do all operations under the low power of the dissecting microscope.

    1. Prepare the necessary number of culture dishes, label them appropriately, and add your initials. Have a dish ready for discarded pieces.

    2. Moisten the cork disk and with the brush place a specimen on it. When the animal is expanded maximally, make a cut with the razor blade in the desired plane. Cut down in a perpendicular direction, not obliquely. The cut surface should be sharp and clean. Practice on several animals before doing the actual experiments.

    3. Take a record and make a sketch.

    4. Transfer the fragment or fragments to the labeled dish and discard the rest of the animal.

    5. Inspect the regenerating pieces every second or third day, depending on the type of experiment. Discard all dead pieces. Indicate clearly on sketches the border line of old and new tissue. Over a long period the regenerating tissue can be distinguished very clearly from the old tissue by its lack of pigmentation. Pay special attention to the first appearance of regenerating eye spots and pharynx. Under ordinary conditions regeneration will be complete in about 8–14 days.

3. REGENERATION AFTER TRANSVERSE, LONGITUDINAL AND OBLIQUE CUTTING

Experiment 57: Regeneration of Transverse Pieces

    Follow the preceding directions. First, decapitate the animal by cutting in plane *a* (Fig. 39, *a*). Next, make section *c,* which is at one-third the length of the decapitated animal.[1] Remove the pharynx if it protrudes. Place each piece in a separate dish; label the dish. Repeat the experiment on 6 animals. Place all identical pieces in the same dish. Make careful observations and sketches of representative cases. Pay special attention to the following points: wound healing; the appearance of the unpigmented regeneration blastema. The head,

[1] Section c is recommended because this cut will serve as a control for Experiment 65. If this experiment is not planned, then make section d (instead of c), which cuts the decapitated animal in half.

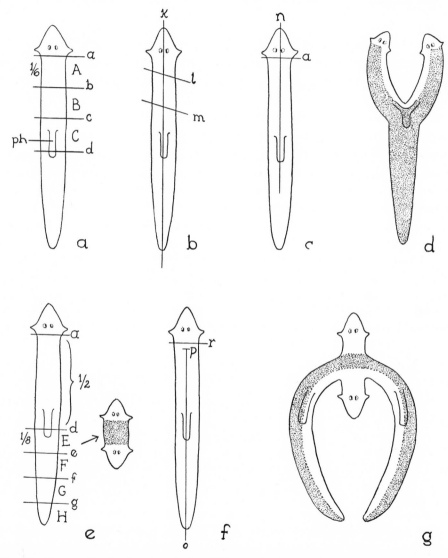

FIG. 39.—Regeneration in planarians (e, from Miller, 1937; f, g, after Silber and Hamburger, 1939). a = different levels of transverse sections; ph = pharynx; b = median (k) and oblique sections (l, m); c, d = production of duplicitas anterior by sectioning in levels a and n; e = production of bipolar forms by regeneration of E-pieces; f, g = production of duplicitas cruciata by sections op and r. The dotted areas in d, e, and g, are old tissue; the light areas in these figures are regenerated tissue.

183

which is characterized by the eye spots, is the first differentiated structure to appear in posterior pieces. It is always formed by blastema cells. Observe the first appearance of the pharynx. It appears near the posterior cut surface in the anterior pieces and near the anterior cut surface in the posterior pieces, usually being formed by old tissue. Note the time required for completion of the regeneration. The end result is in each instance a smaller but proportionate individual. The original polarity is maintained in all fragments. Any level is capable of forming a head.

Experiment 58: Regeneration of Short Transverse Pieces

Make a transection behind the head (Fig. 39, *a*, level *a*) and bisect the body (level *d*). Cut the anterior half in 3 (one-sixth) or 4 (one-eighth) pieces of equal lengths and keep all pieces of the same level in one dish. Label the dishes. Operate 6 animals. In this experiment study mainly the attainment of the typical proportions by the formation of blastemas as well as by morphallaxis. All short pieces are at the beginning much too wide as compared to their lengths. The heads (old or regenerated) will at first be disproportionately large. Note the gradual adjustments of the proportions by changes in shape. Note again the regeneration of a new pharynx, usually in the old tissue. The head malformations that occur frequently in short transverse pieces are discussed on page 187 (see Fig. 40).

Experiment 59: Lateral Regeneration

Section several planarians in the median plane (*k*, Fig. 39, *b*). Section others in a paramedian plane. Discard all pieces of the old pharynx. Observe lateral regeneration.

Experiment 60: Regeneration from Oblique Surfaces

Make an oblique cut and discard the anterior piece. In another series make two parallel oblique cuts in the prepharyngeal region (*l* and *m*, Fig. 39, *b*); discard head and posterior end. Note that the head regenerating at the anterior surface makes its appearance not in the middle of the cut surface but at its most anterior point. It is asymmetrical at first. This asymmetry is clearly expressed in the earlier appearance of the left (anterior) eye. The tail blastema is likewise asymmetrical. The regenerates illustrate another point of general interest: the main direction of outgrowth both of head and of tail blastemas is at first perpendicular to the cut surface and not in the main axis of the old piece. In later stages the heads and tails straighten out. Rulon (1936) has interpreted these results on the basis of Child's gradient theory.

4. PRODUCTION OF TWO-HEADED PLANARIANS
(DUPLICITAS ANTERIOR)

EXPERIMENT 61

Remove the head behind the eyes (a, Fig. 39, c) and split the anterior two-thirds of the animal in the median line (n). The separated parts have a strong tendency to heal together, and if necessary the slit must be reopened several times within 12–24 hours. Note the appearance of new eyes and new pharynges. The experiment shows that the regenerate of a planaria behaves like a 2-cell stage of a salamander or of a sea-urchin egg. Each half tends to reconstitute a whole organism (Fig. 39, d).

4a. PRODUCTION OF TWO-TAILED PLANARIANS
(DUPLICITAS POSTERIOR)

EXPERIMENT 62

Remove the head behind the eyes and split the posterior two-thirds of the animal. Two tails will form if the parts are kept separate by continued reopening of the slit.

5. PRODUCTION OF BIPOLAR FORMS
(POLAR HETEROMORPHOSES)

The previous experiments have given evidence that the polarity is usually maintained in regenerating planarians. Cases in which the polarity is changed are therefore of special interest. Morgan was the first to describe the regeneration of two heads from the anterior and the posterior cut surfaces of a short transverse piece; he called this phenomenon "heteromorphosis." Later on, the term was used to designate all kinds of atypical regenerations, for instance, the regeneration of antennae in the place of amputated eye stalks in arthropods. To avoid confusion, inversions of polarity are now called "polar heteromorphoses." They occur occasionally after transverse section immediately behind the eyes or in very short transverse pieces of post-pharyngeal levels. Their incidence can be increased by various agents, such as ether, chloretone, or strychnine.[2] The following experiment is based on the strychnine experiment of F. S. Miller (1937).

These polar heteromorphoses are usually explained in terms of the gradient theory. It is assumed that the physiological activity at the 2 surfaces is so

[2] H. Kanatani (Jour. Fac. Sci. Univ. of Tokyo, Sec. IV, 8:253) using *Dugesia gonocephala,* obtained a high percentage of bipolar heads by treatment of the whole animals with Demecolcine ("Colcemide," deacetylmethylcolchicine, Ciba) preceding the cutting. A stock solution was prepared containing 0.1% demecolcine, 10% propylene glycol, and 5% ethanol. This solution was diluted M/7,590–M/30,000 and the animals kept in different concentrations for 48 hours before sectioning. Temperatures of 22°–25° C. were found to be optimal. The animals were then washed, decapitated, and the anterior halves cut into 3 or 4 pieces of equal length (i.e., 1/6 or 1/8 pieces) and reared in well or pond water.

nearly equal that no metabolic gradient is set up between them; hence, neither exerts physiological dominance over the other, and both proceed with head formation simultaneously. However, this may be an oversimplification. The conditions for regeneration in very short pieces may be atypical in other respects. For instance, in longer pieces an agent inhibiting head formation is activated at the posterior cut surface (see Experiment 66, p. 190). This agent, which is supposedly produced by the nerve cords, may not be formed in very short pieces.

(see Experiment 66, p. 190)

Experiment 63

Material

Dugesia dorotocephala, 10–15 specimens per student

other material as on page 182

prepare a fresh solution of strychnine sulphate, M/100,000, for each experiment

Procedure

Make all sections in water, not in the strychnine solution. For the following experiments only post-pharyngeal one-eighth pieces will be used. E-pieces (Fig. 39, e) give the highest percentage of bipolar heads. F-pieces may also be used. Cut in the following order: a, d, f, e (Fig. 39, e). Discard all but the E- and F-pieces. Transfer these fragments immediately to the strychnine solution, cover the dishes, and keep them in a dark, cool place. After 12–16 hours transfer all pieces to spring or well water. A longer exposure is lethal. Check the cultures frequently and remove dead fragments. Observe the development of bipolar forms. Atypical heads (see p. 188, Fig. 40) will be found occasionally. Note the direction of the beat of cilia (cf. Miller, 1937). The percentage of bipolar heads can be increased further by delaying the posterior cut for 12–24 hours. Run parallel cultures of E- and F-pieces in well or spring water as controls.

6. PRODUCTION OF DUPLICITAS CRUCIATA

Experiment 64

Duplicitas cruciata is one of the strangest duplications occurring in animals. It is a complete duplication in which two heads and two tails are present. The two heads face in opposite directions and have a common median plane; likewise the two tails point in opposite directions. However, the median planes of the heads and of the tails are perpendicular to each other (Fig. 39, g). For details concerning the following experiment see Silber and Hamburger (1939).

Material

Dugesia tigrina, or D. dorotocephala, 10 specimens per student

other material as on p. 182

Procedure (see p. 182)

Make a longitudinal cut in the median plane through body and tail to a point behind the auricles (*o–p* in Fig. 39, *f*). After 24 hours make a transverse cut (*r*) at a short distance in front of the crotch, so that the two half-tails are held together by a narrow connection about one-third their width. If necessary, reopen the longitudinal cut. Make 6–10 operations. Check the operated animals on the following days. Reopen the median slit whenever necessary.

In a high percentage of cases the anterior transverse surface will regenerate a normal head, and another normal head will develop in the crotch (Fig. 39, *g*). The crotch heads are occasionally duplicated or abnormal. The anterior heads are either normal or, in a few cases, absent. Observe the movements of these monsters after completion of the regeneration. Either head may take the lead, with the other head and the tails trailing behind, and they may alternate in leading.

7. THE INFLUENCE OF THE AXIAL GRADIENT ON HEAD REGENERATION IN PLANARIA

HEAD FREQUENCY

Child and his school have widely used "head frequency" as a convenient semiquantitative measure for the influence of the axial gradient and depressing chemical agents on regeneration in planarians. Head frequency expresses the percentage of normal head regenerates, taking into account the number and degree of abnormal head regenerates that are found under special experimental conditions. The head regenerates can be arranged in a graded series, ranging from normal heads to small outgrowths. They were classified by Child in five arbitrary groups (see Fig. 40): I. Normal. II. Teratophthalmic (abnormal eyes). The shape of the head is almost normal, but the eyes show all degrees of approximation and fusion to the point of cyclopia (one single eye). We have included in this group the cases in which one eye is normal and the other small. III. Teratomorphic (abnormal head). The shape of the head is abnormal, and there is usually only one eye present. IV. Anophthalmic (eyeless). The shape of the head is abnormal, usually to a higher degree than in III, and the eyes are not formed. V. Acephalic (no head). In extreme cases no head regenerates at the anterior end (further details in Child, 1941, pp. 171 ff.).

In order to obtain a statistical measure of the degree of head inhibition in a mass experiment, arbitrary numerical values were assigned to these five classes, namely, I $= 100$, II $= 80$, III $= 60$, IV $= 40$, V $= 20$. The head frequency is calculated after the formula

$$\text{h. fr.} = \frac{100 \cdot n_{\text{I}} + 80 \cdot n_{\text{II}} + 60 \cdot n_{\text{III}} + 40 \cdot n_{\text{IV}} + 20 \cdot n_{\text{V}}}{n},$$

where n_{I}–n_{V} are the numbers of cases of the different types of heads and n is the total number of surviving animals. It should be emphasized that the head-

187

frequency value thus obtained is not an exact mean head frequency in the statistical sense, because the numerical values are entirely arbitrary. The head-frequency figures are useful only as a convenient means of comparing the degree of head inhibition under different experimental conditions (see Child, 1941, p. 745; also Castle, 1940).

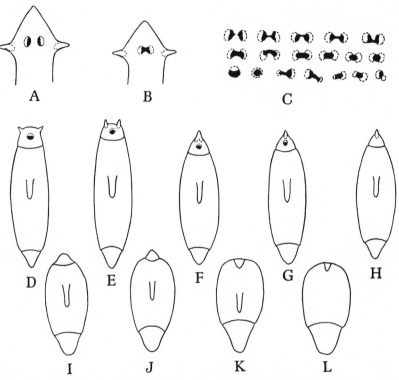

FIG. 40.—The inhibition series of head forms of *D. (Pl.) dorotocephala* (from Child, 1941). *A* = normal head; *B* = teratophthalmic head; *C* = eyes of teratophthalmic heads; *D–G* = teratomorphic heads; *H–J* = anophthalmic heads; *K, L* = acephalic forms.

Example.—In a lot of 20 pieces we find 5 normal, 7 teratophthalmic, 3 teratomorphic, 3 anophthalmic, and 2 acephalic specimens:

$$\text{h. fr.} = \frac{5 \cdot 100 + 7 \cdot 80 + 3 \cdot 60 + 3 \cdot 40 + 2 \cdot 20}{20} = 70.$$

The following experiment is based on Child and Watanabe (1935). It is supposed to illustrate a basic point of the gradient theory, namely, the influence of axial gradients on differentiation processes. It will be found that short transverse pieces from anterior levels have a higher head frequency than do pieces from posterior levels, all other factors being equal.

188

Material

Dugesia (*Pl.*) *dorotocephala*, 15–20 specimens per student (They should be of as uniform size as possible, approximately 14–18 mm. in length.)

other material; see p. 182

Procedure (*see p. 182*)

1. Fill 3 finger bowls or paraffined paper cups with pond or spring water; label them A, B, C.

2. Select 15 healthy specimens of as uniform size as possible. Place a specimen on a moistened cork disk under the binocular microscope, using the brush for transfer.

3. Amputate the head immediately behind the eyes (level *a*, Fig. 39, *a*) and discard it.

4. Allow the animal to stretch maximally and cut it exactly in two halves (level *d*, Fig. 39, *a*). Discard the posterior half.[3]

5. Allow the anterior half to stretch and cut it into three equal parts (levels

No. OPER-ATED	DIED	HEAD FORMS						RESULTS OF CLASS	
		I	II	III	IV	V	Head Frequency	Number Operated	Head Frequency
A......									
B......									
C......									

b and *c*, Fig. 39, *a*). Discard all parts of specimens which were not cut equally. Do not use the pharynx as a landmark. If the pharynx is extruded, remove it altogether.

Repeat the experiment with 10–14 other animals.

6. Transfer all anterior one-sixth pieces to the dish labeled A, all middle pieces to dish B, and all posterior pieces to dish C. Take a record. Place the dishes in a cool, dark place.

7. After 2 days remove the dead fragments. Do not feed.

8. Study the regenerates 10–14 days after operation. Inspect each lot separately. Make sketches of representative specimens of the five head types. If not all are represented in your material, exchange specimens with other students. Determine the numbers of the different head forms in each lot and tabulate the results as in the accompanying table. Add the total figures for the class and plot them as a curve.

[3] Posterior halves will not be used in this experiment, in order to avoid complications which arise from the occurrence of fission (asexual reproduction by transverse division of animals). The planes of fission are anticipated by a local rise in metabolic activity, which distorts the axial gradient in the posterior half.

1. Compare head frequency in pieces A, B, and C of the present experiment. The only variable is the body level. What conclusion can be drawn?

2. Compare head frequency in C-pieces with that in tail pieces of Experiment 57 (p. 182). The only variable in the two experiments is the length of the piece. What conclusion can be drawn? (See the following experiment.)

8. DELAYED POSTERIOR SECTIONS

This experiment should be done in conjunction with the preceding experiment. It carries the analysis of head determination one step further. Child and Watanabe (1935) and Watanabe (1935) performed a variety of experiments of partial or total transection, in which the length of the piece was varied and the anterior and posterior cuts were made either simultaneously or at different time intervals. The results indicate that an inhibitory factor is activated by the posterior cut; that it is produced or transmitted by the nerve cords, with a decrement in posterior–anterior direction; and that it exerts its depressing effect on head differentiation within 8–12 hours after cutting (in *D. dorotocephala*).

We have selected an experiment of delayed posterior section which gives evidence for the last-mentioned point. It was demonstrated previously (Exp. 57, p. 182) that level *c* (Fig. 39, *a*) produces 100 per cent normal heads, under normal environmental conditions, if no other cut is made posterior to *c*, but that a certain percentage of abnormal heads are formed, that is, the "head frequency" is lowered, if cut *d* is made a short distance from *c* (see preceding experiment). By delaying the posterior cut for increasing time intervals, one finds that the head frequency increases steadily until it reaches 100 per cent at a delay of 8–12 hours (in *D. dorotocephala;* earlier in *D. maculata*). This implies that the inhibitory agent influences the head determination in very early stages of blastema formation.

EXPERIMENT 66

Material

Dugesia (Pl.) dorotocephala or D. tigrina; 15–30 specimens for each student (Select individuals of uniform size.)

other material as in Experiment 65

Procedure (see p. 182)

1. Cut all specimens in the *c*-level (Fig. 39, *a*) and discard all anterior pieces.

2. Make cuts in level *d:*

a) in 5–10 specimens, 2 hours after cut *c*

b) in 5–10 specimens, 8–14 hours after cut *c*

c) in 5–10 specimens, 24 hours after cut *c*

190

Discard the posterior pieces. Keep the 3 lots in different dishes and handle the material as in Experiment 65.

3. After 2 weeks, calculate the head frequency for the 3 series, as in Experiment 65. Tabulate and plot the results on graph paper. Compare your curves with those of Child and Watanabe (1935) for *D. dorotocephala* and Watanabe (1935) for *D. tigrina*. Note that these authors worked with one-eighth and one-tenth pieces. Temperature and other conditions may also have an effect on the results.

BIBLIOGRAPHY

BRONDSTED, H. V. 1955. Planarian regeneration. Biol. Rev., **30**:65.

CASTLE, W. A. 1940. Methods for evaluation of head types in planarians. Physiol. Zoöl., **13**:309.

CHILD, C. M. 1941. Patterns and problems of development. Chicago: University of Chicago Press.

———— and WATANABE, Y. 1935. The head frequency gradient in *Euplanaria dorotocephala*. Physiol. Zoöl., **8**:1.

HYMAN, L. 1931. Studies on the morphology, taxonomy, and distribution of North American Triclad Turbellaria. IV. Trans. Amer. Micr. Soc., **50**:316.

————. 1937. Planarians. In GALTSOFF, P. S. (ed.), Culture methods for invertebrate animals. Ithaca, N.Y.: Comstock Pub. Co.

KORSCHELT, E. 1927. Regeneration und Transplantation, Vol. **1**. Berlin: Borntraeger.

MILLER, F. S. 1937. Some effects of strychnine on reconstitution in *Euplanaria dorotocephala*. Physiol. Zoöl., **10**:276.

RULON, O. 1936. Experimental asymmetries of the head of *Euplanaria dorotocephala*. Physiol. Zoöl., **9**:278.

SILBER, R. H., and HAMBURGER, V. 1939. The production of duplicitas cruciata and multiple heads by regeneration in *Euplanaria tigrina*. Physiol. Zoöl., **12**:285.

WATANABE, Y. 1935. Head frequency in *Euplanaria maculata* in relation to the nervous system. Physiol. Zoöl., **8**:374.

C. REGENERATION IN AMPHIBIAN LARVAE

1. TAIL REGENERATION

Tail regeneration in anuran tadpoles and in larval and adult urodeles is one of the best known examples of regeneration. Larvae will be used in the following experiments because the regeneration of adult salamander tails takes several months.

There are considerable structural differences between the tails of frog tadpoles and of salamander larvae; they reflect the divergence of the two groups since their early evolutionary history. The tadpole tail lacks vertebrae, and the somewhat enlarged notochord is its only skeletal reinforcement; whereas vertebrae with neural and hemal arches are present in salamander larvae. The regenerated tails of both groups appear outwardly to be complete, but those of the salamander are structurally deficient in that the notochord fails to regenerate. It is replaced functionally by a series of segmented cartilages in the position of the notochord; they are precociously differentiated vertebral centra (H. Holtzer and others, 1955). The frog tadpoles regenerate all axial organs, including the notochord.

Following amputation, a "blastema," or regeneration bud, is formed; it is composed of undifferentiated mesenchyme-like cells covered by epithelium. Its main axis is perpendicular to the cut surface. If an oblique cut is made, the blastema grows out at an angle to the main axis but straightens out later ("functional adaptation"). Although our experiments afford no opportunity to study the mode of differentiation of the regenerating axial organs and the role of the blastema in this process, we shall discuss these questions briefly because they touch on central problems in Vertebrate regeneration.

The origin of regenerating structures in urodeles has been a matter of intense investigations and dispute. According to one extreme view, each structure is formed by outgrowth from its own type of tissue at the amputation surface; according to another view, the regenerating structures differentiate from indifferent blastema cells. The tail-regeneration process is a combination of both. There is no doubt that the spinal cord, and in anuran tadpoles the notochord, are formed by direct outgrowth of the old structures in the stump. It is less easy to prove, but well substantiated, that the regeneration of the tail musculature takes the same course. Muscles near the cut surface dedifferentiate and partly redifferentiate into myoblasts with single nuclei, which form new muscles in continuity with those of the stump.

On the other hand, the cartilage in the regenerating salamander tail is probably derived entirely from blastema cells (S. Holtzer, 1956). This raises the question of the origin of the blastema. The major source of the blastema cell material seems to be the musculature of the stump. Whereas part of the small cells with single nuclei that bud off from intact muscle fibers at the amputation surface redifferentiate into muscle, others assume the form of mesenchyme-like cells and enter the blastema. Connective tissue cells from the stump probably contribute also to the blastema. Since the vertebral cartilage is formed by blastema cells, it is implied that one type of tissue, namely muscle, can be transformed into another type, namely cartilage, after it has gone through a transitional, undifferentiated stage. Such a transformation of fully differentiated tissue is called "metaplasia." We shall encounter another instance in lens regeneration (p. 197). The importance of metaplasia for the general problem of differentiation and its reversibility is obvious. It is of interest to note that this particular metaplastic transformation into cartilage requires an inductive stimulus from the spinal cord (S. Holtzer, 1956).

Experiment 67

Material

    Ambystoma or *Triturus* or *Rana,* any species (stages from swimming stages on)

1 pair of fine forceps	Petri dishes
1 pair of fine scissors, preferably iridectomy scissors (p. 9).	chloretone 1:3,000, or MS 222, 1:5,000 for narcosis (do not narcotize frog tadpoles; see pp. 40,
pipettes	cotize frog tadpoles; see pp. 40,
finger bowls or paper cups	135)

Procedure

1. Narcotize 10 specimens of equal size (take measurements). Operate in narcotic in Petri dishes.

2. With a pair of fine scissors amputate the tails. In 5 specimens make the cuts transversely. In 5 specimens make them obliquely. Record the details of the operation. Make sketches of representative cases.

3. Feed the animals daily (p. 26).

4. Observe the wound-healing and the daily progress of regeneration, the appearance of the blastema, its outgrowth, the differentiation of the fins, pigmentation, etc. Observe in particular the direction of outgrowth in the obliquely cut animals. The angle between the main axis of the animal and the axis of the regenerating tail can be observed best during the first days after the appearance of the blastema. Later on, the regenerating tip straightens out.

2. LIMB REGENERATION

Urodeles in larval and adult stages can regenerate a limb after amputation at any level, even after complete extirpation of the limb and girdle (see p. 178).

In anurans, the legs regenerate only in larval stages. Occasionally the regenerates are atypical; for instance, the number of toes may be reduced (hypodactyly) or increased (hyperdactyly). Duplications are of particular interest because they give evidence that the early regeneration blastema is not a mosaic but has regulative properties.

Amputation is followed by epidermal wound closure and a dedifferentiation process that involves the mesodermal tissues near the amputation surface, especially musculature and skeletal elements (see Butler, 1933; Nicholas, 1955). This regression soon comes to a halt, and the formation of a typical blastema sets in. The questions raised above (p. 192) in connection with tail regeneration are also pertinent with respect to limb regeneration. It seems that regeneration by direct outgrowth of old tissue plays a less important role here than in tail regeneration and that it is limited to nerve and epidermis outgrowth. Skeletal differentiation in the regenerate does not depend on the presence of skeletal elements at the amputation surface. This can be demonstrated experimentally by carefully dissecting out a skeletal element—for instance, the humerus—and amputating subsequently in the middle of the upper arm. The humerus is not replaced, but the regenerate distal to it contains a normal skeleton (Weiss, 1925, and others). Hence, skeleton, and probably also musculature, can differentiate from the blastema.

Despite extensive investigation, the question of the origin of the blastema cells is not definitely solved because of the difficulty of tracing the cells of the stump. During the regressive phase which follows amputation, both dedifferentiated muscle cells and dedifferentiated skeletal cells seem to be transformed into mesenchyme-like cells which contribute to the blastema. Connective tissue cells of the stump and perhaps epidermis are other sources for blastema cells. It seems unlikely that the individual blastema cells retain their original tissue specificity. Rather, the cells which form the early blastema seem to be pluripotent, and true metaplasia (see p. 193) is a definite possibility.

PRELIMINARY EXERCISE

In order to find out whether the development of the external form of regenerates proceeds along the same lines as does normal limb development, study the development of normal forelimbs in *Ambystoma* (any species). Start out with 3–5 larvae of stage H40 and make a complete series of sketches up to stages in which all digits are formed. Narcotize the animals during observations. Note in particular the appearance of the elbow, the sequence of the appearance of the digits, and their relative proportions. Take notes on the rate of differentiation under the temperature and other conditions of your experiment. The animals should be kept at a constant temperature if possible.

Material

    Ambystoma larvae with 4 digits, 4–6 specimens for each student. Select specimens whose limbs and toes are completely intact. When several specimens are kept in the same dish, they frequently injure each other's limbs, particularly if they are not fed adequately. It is therefore advisable to rear the specimens to be used in this experiment singly in paraffined paper cups or glass dishes.

1 pair of fine forceps	a dish with wax bottom
1 pair of fine scissors, preferably iridectomy scissors (p. 9)	pipettes
	chloretone 1:3,000 or MS 222
finger bowls or paraffined paper cups	1:5,000 for narcosis

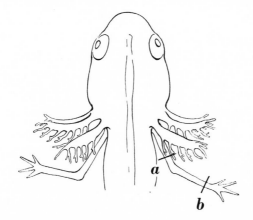

Fig. 41.—Forelimb regeneration in urodele larva. *a, b* = levels of amputation (see text)

Procedure

    1. Narcotize 4–5 specimens.

    2. Make a sketch of the extended right arm of a representative specimen. Use the camera lucida if available. In order to mount the arm horizontally, use a dish with wax bottom. Make a deep groove in which the body of the animal fits and spread the arm over the edge of the groove.

    3. In 2–3 specimens make a transverse cut through the right humerus (Fig. 41, *a*); in 2–3 specimens amputate the right hand through the wrist (*b*). Use a pair of fine scissors. Indicate the level of cutting on the sketch.

    4. Give each specimen a serial number and place each in a separate dish. Rear animals at constant temperature if possible.

    5. Follow the regeneration for several weeks. Make a complete series of sketches. Compare the regeneration with normal development. Note that in the specimens amputated at the humerus the digits will appear first and the parts between the digits and the cut level will be restored later. If time per-

mits, both the amputated ends and the fully regenerated limbs should be fixed and stained with methylene blue (van Wijhe method, see below), in order to find out whether the cartilaginous skeleton has been restored completely.

3. A MODIFIED VAN WIJHE STAIN FOR CARTILAGE[4]

The following procedure is recommended for the staining of the cartilage of regenerated and control limbs of amphibian larvae. It is a modification of the method of van Wijhe (Proc. Roy. Acad. Sci. Amsterdam, **5**:45, 1902), devised by V. Gregg and E. G. Butler of Princeton University.

Fixative:

Formalin (40 per cent)	5 cc.
Alcohol (70 per cent)	95 cc.

Methylene blue stain:

Methylene blue	0.25 grams
Alcohol (70 per cent)	100 cc.
Hydrochloric acid	0.5 cc.

Procedure

1. Fix in formol-alcohol, 24 hours or longer. May be left in fixative indefinitely.

2. Without washing, transfer material into the stain for 10–60 minutes, depending on the size and thickness of the specimen.

3. Without washing, transfer specimen directly to 95 per cent alcohol for destaining. The alcohol must be changed as it becomes colored. This must be done very carefully by gently tapping the specimen with a curved needle or a blunt and rounded glass rod until no more color comes away in clouds visible under the binocular microscope.

4. Dehydrate in absolute alcohol, three changes in 45 minutes, at 15-minute intervals.

5. Clear in methyl salicylate (synthetic) U.S.P. (oil of wintergreen). May be left in this clearing agent indefinitely.

6. Whole mounts are prepared by transferring the specimen to xylol for 10–60 minutes to wash off excess methyl salicylate.

7. Take a clean slide, put a drop of Damarbalsam on the spot where the specimen is to be fastened (for a base). Allow the balsam to "set" 10–30 minutes in an oven or over a warm plate at 50°–60° C. temperature.

8. Transfer the specimen onto the spot and add layers of balsam at 2–4-hour intervals until the specimen is completely covered with the balsam, and leave over night at the same temperature.

9. On the following day the specimen should be fully infiltrated with the balsam, which should be quite firm. Another layer of the mounting medium

---

[4] I am greatly indebted to Dr. E. G. Butler, who made the unpublished account of this method available to me.

should be added, and the specimen covered with a cover glass. The completed preparation should be set aside to harden.

Results

Cartilaginous skeleton and bone blue; all other tissues colorless or faintly colored.

4. LENS REGENERATION IN URODELES

The remarkable regenerative capacity of urodeles extends to the crystalline lens of the eye. If the lens is extirpated in a larval or adult salamander or newt, it will regenerate from the upper iris. The iris is an epithelial pigmented double layer, folded upon itself. In regeneration, its dorsal margin becomes depigmented and grows out to form a vesicle which is suspended in the pupil; it differentiates lens fibers and eventually detaches from the iris and assumes the regular lens position behind the pupil. The process is described in detail and illustrated in Reyer (1954) and Dinnean (1942). The frequently used term "Wolffian lens regeneration" refers to G. Wolff, a German zoölogist and neurologist who made the first extensive analysis of lens regeneration, around the turn of the century.

The phenomenon of lens regeneration exhibits a number of unusual features. For instance, the origin of the regenerated lens is different from that of the embryonic lens, which is derived from the epidermis overlying the optic vesicle (see p. 114). It is remarkable that two very different developmental pathways can lead to identical end products. Furthermore, this is one of the few clear cases of "metaplasia," that is, the dedifferentiation of a differentiated tissue, the pigmented iris epithelium, and its redifferentiation to form another highly specialized structure (see p. 193).

Lens regeneration deviates from other regeneration processes in one respect: In most instances the regeneration process is set in motion by the creation of a wound surface. If the lens extirpation experiment is done carefully, however, there is no injury to the upper iris. What, then, is the activating stimulus in this case? We know that lens regeneration does not start unless the lens is removed, which points to an inhibitory effect of the lens. There is evidence to show that the lens exerts this influence not by mechanical pressure on the upper iris but by the release of a chemical agent into the aqueous humor. If aqueous humor from an eye with lens is injected in the posterior chamber of an eye from which the lens has been removed, regeneration does not take place (Stone, 1959). It is likely, however, that the removal of this inhibitor alone is not sufficient to activate the regeneration process. It seems that another agent, produced by the retina, the so-called "retina factor," plays an imporant role as activator or inductor of lens regeneration. It is assumed that the retina factor is inhibited as long as the lens is present and that it begins to stimulate the upper iris as soon as the lens is extirpated (see Reyer, 1954; Stone, 1959).

The capacity for lens regeneration is not restricted to the upper margin of the iris. Tests for lens competence were done in an experiment in which small pieces from different areas of the iris were implanted in the posterior chamber of a lensless eye, where they proceeded to regenerate. In this way it was found that the regenerative capacity has its peak at the dorsal margin and declines toward the equator; it is practically absent at the ventral margin (Sato, 1930). The upper and lateral margins of the iris represent a lens-regeneration *gradient-field*.

The capacity for lens regeneration seems to be restricted to *Urodela* (the few data on anurans are inconclusive), and even among this group one finds considerable differences. Lens regeneration occurs rather regularly in all species of the genera *Triturus* and *Taricha* throughout life, but it is much more erratic in *Ambystoma*. In our class experiments we observed over a period of several years lens regeneration in *A. opacum* and *maculatum;* but the number of successful cases was variable and never exceeded 50 per cent. It is recommended that *Ambystoma* larvae be used only if the other species are not available and that in this case a larger number of experiments be done than is suggested below.

Although adults of *Triturus* and *Taricha* can perform lens regeneration, medium-sized or older larvae are obviously the material of choice: the operation, handling, and rearing are simpler. Data on speed of regeneration may be found in Reyer (1954). A period of 4–5 weeks should be allowed for this experiment.

EXPERIMENT 69

Material

Larvae of *Triturus* or *Taricha*, with 3 toes or older; if these are not available, then *Ambystoma*, stage H46 or older; six or more specimens per student

steel knife with very sharp point (prepared by sharpening the point of a sewing needle, see p. 9)

glass needle, straight, not elastic, tapering into a fine point

1 pair of forceps

operation dishes with wax bottom

medium-size paraffined paper cups for rearing of larvae

filter paper, insect pins

chloretone 1:3,000 or MS 222 1:5,000 for narcosis

Procedure

1. Prepare a groove in the wax bottom of the operating dish, deep enough to hold the larva when lying on its side. Prepare broad strips of filter paper to hold the larva in the groove; pierce the ends with insect pins while paper is dry.

2. Narcotize 3–4 larvae at a time.

3. Fill the operation dish with narcotic. Place the larva in the groove, right side up, and pin it down tightly with the strip of filter paper.

4. Hold the head down with a pair of forceps. Pierce the cornea on one side of the lens with the sharp point of the steel knife and enlarge the hole by cutting until the lens is completely exposed (Fig. 42, *a*). Avoid injury to the darkly pigmented iris. Sometimes, a slight pressure on the eye with the forceps forces the lens out. If not, lift the lens out with the tip of the steel knife or of the glass needle, inserted between the rim of the pupil and the lens. The extirpated lens is visible as a glass-clear spherical body. In each case it should be ascertained that the lens was actually removed intact; small fragments of the lens which are left behind can regenerate a lens and thus invalidate the experiment. Discard specimens in which the lens was torn during the operation. Avoid

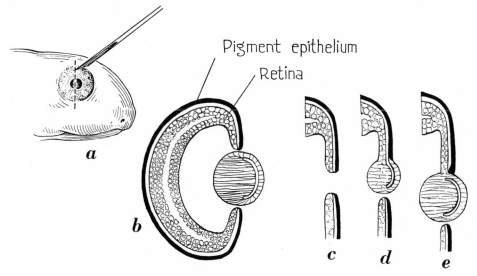

Fig. 42.—Lens-regeneration experiment in urodeles. *a* = operation (see text). The cornea is cut along the dotted line. *b* = normal eye; *c* = iris after lens extirpation; *d, e* = stages of lens regeneration from the upper iris.

hemorrhage and damage to the iris or retina. Discard cases in which the retina, a whitish material, protrudes from the wound.

This manipulation requires some practice. Use both eyes of one or two specimens for practicing.

5. Make 6–10 operations. Take a record and place each individual in a separate dish. Note that the pupil contracts after the operation.

6. Make a check of all operated specimens 8–10 days after the operation, and from then on at shorter intervals. Note the gradual reopening of the pupil. Under strong illumination and high magnification, the formation of a small vesicle at the upper iris can observed. In general, the gradual widening of the pupil gives an indication of the progression of the regeneration process. Feed

animals well and keep them in isolation. In medium-sized larvae, the regeneration should be completed within 4 weeks.

7. Terminate the experiment after 4–5 weeks. Narcotize all specimens and fix them in 10 per cent formaldehyde. After a few minutes, the lenses become opaque and very distinct. Wash the animals in water and dissect the skin from over both eyes. If a camera lucida is available, make drawings of the contours of lens and eye on both sides and calculate the eye-lens index = ratio of eye diameter to lens diameter. Compare the ratios for the normal and the operated eye.

8. The results of the class should be tabulated as follows and the percentages calculated.

No. oper.	No. survived	Lens of normal or near n. size	Small lens	No. regeneration

If facilities are available, a number of experimental animals should be sacrificed at intervals, between 5 and 25 days after operation, for microscopic study of intermediate stages. (See illustrations for *Triturus viridescens* in Reyer (1954) and for *Taricha torosa* in Dinnean (1942).

BIBLIOGRAPHY

BUTLER, E. G. 1933. The effects of X-radiation on the regeneration of the forelimb of *Amblystoma* larvae. Jour. Exper. Zool., **65**:271.

DINNEAN, F. L. 1942. Lens regeneration from the iris and its inhibition by lens reimplantation in *Triturus torosus* larvae. Jour. Exper. Zool., **90**:461–78.

HOLTZER, H., HOLTZER, S., and AVERY, G. 1955. An experimental analysis of the development of the spinal column. IV. Morphogenesis of tail vertebrae during regeneration. Jour. Morphol., **96**:145–72.

HOLTZER, S. 1956. The inductive activity of the spinal cord in urodele tail regeneration. Jour. Morphol., **99**:1–40.

NICHOLAS, J. S. 1955. Regeneration, vertebrates. In WILLIER, WEISS, and HAMBURGER (eds.), Analysis of development. Philadelphia: Saunders.

REYER, R. W. 1954. Regeneration of the lens in the amphibian eye. Quart. Rev. Biol., **29**:1–41.

SATO, TADAO. 1930. Beiträge zur Analyse der Wolff'schen Linsenregeneration. I. Arch. f. Entw'mech., **122**:451–92.

STONE, L. S. 1959. Regeneration of the retina, iris, and lens. In THORNTON (ed.), Regeneration in vertebrates. Chicago: University of Chicago Press.

WEISS, P. 1925. Unabhängigkeit der Extremitätenregeneration vom Skelett. Arch. f. mikr. Anat. u. Entw'mech., **104**:359.

APPENDIX

PLAN FOR A ONE-SEMESTER COURSE

A course in experimental embryology requires of the instructor a great deal of advanced planning, continuous attention to the individual students during the laboratory periods and at extra hours, and resourcefulness in cases of emergencies, which are hardly avoidable when one relies on supply with living embryos. For these and other reasons it is advisable to limit the class to 12–15 students.

As stated in the Introduction, the experiments are arranged according to topics and concepts and not in the order in which they should be performed. The planning of the course is left to the discretion and preferences of the instructor. In designing the course, several important points have to be taken into consideration. Much depends on the availability of amphibian material which is the "backbone" of the course. Frog eggs can now be obtained at almost any season by induced ovulation, and they can be used for a variety of experiments; yet, *Ambystoma* is the material of choice for some of the most attractive experiments, such as transplantation and vital staining. The breeding season of *A. punctatum* is from the end of January to February in southern locations, March and April in the Middle West, and April to May in northern regions. *A. opacum* is available in September and October. In our own course (spring semester), we use *Ambystoma* from the beginning of the semester through March, frog embryos in March and part of April, salamander larvae raised by the students and planarians for regeneration experiments in April and May, and chick embryos during the last weeks.

Another question requires some thought: how to introduce the novice effectively to the art of handling the living embryos and to the delicate operational procedures. One would want to start out with experiments which are not too difficult, yet challenging the skill and rewarding. I have found that most students are sufficiently skilful to master such experiments as balancer transplantation or parabiosis without much previous experience, when properly instructed. As was pointed out above (p. 41), the preparation of appropriate instruments (glass needles, etc.) exactly according to specifications is an absolutely necessary prerequisite.

At the beginning of our course all students do the same experiments; later on, smaller groups may be assigned different experiments, and the results demonstrated to the class. Some of the experiments are too difficult to be assigned to the class; they should be demonstrated by the instructor. In the following, the major experiments are listed in three groups, according to the skill required to perform them:

Easy: 4–7, 8, 10, 20–22, 23, 30, 38, 42–45, 57–62, 65, 67–68.
More difficult but suitable as classroom experiment: 1–3, 12, 15, 19, 27, 34, 37, 41, 50–52, 53, 63, 64, 69.
Difficult; requiring considerable experience: 9, 11, 39, 40, 47–49, 54–56.

Following is the list of experiments from which I select in planning our own one-semester course. We accomplish approximately two-thirds of the experiments, with some variations each year. The experiments are listed approximately in the order in which they are scheduled. A = *Ambystoma,* F = frog; the numbers in parentheses refer to experiments in the text.

Normal development of *Ambystoma*
Preparation of instruments (pp. 3 ff.)
Balancer (limb, eye, gill) transplantations (A, 12, 15, 19)
Extirpation of eye primordia in neurula and tail-bud stages (A, 30, 34, 36, 37)
Removal of prospective lens epithelium (A, F, 38)
Extirpation of parts of the limb field (A, 23)
Vital staining in the gastrula and neurula (A, 1–6)
Vital staining of the lateral-line primordia (A, *Taricha;* 7)
Exogastrulation (A, 43)
Parabiosis (A, F,41)
Heart duplications (A, 27)
Isolation experiments (A, F, 20–22)
Origin of behavior (A, 45, 46)
Induced ovulation and artificial insemination (F, p. 28)
Artificial parthenogenesis (F, 8)
Diverse experiments on tail-bud stages (F)
Regeneration of limbs (A, 68) and tails (A, F, 67)
Lens regeneration (*Taricha,* 69)
Planarian regeneration (selectd from 57–64; 65 always being included)
Lithium experiments (F, 42)
Thyroxin experiments (F, 44)
Chorio-allantoic grafts (50–52)
Vital staining in chick embryo (47–49)
Coelomic grafts in chick embryo (53)
Demonstrations
Androgenetic haploidy (F, 9)
Organizer experiments (A, 39, or 40)
Transplantations in chick embryo (54–56)

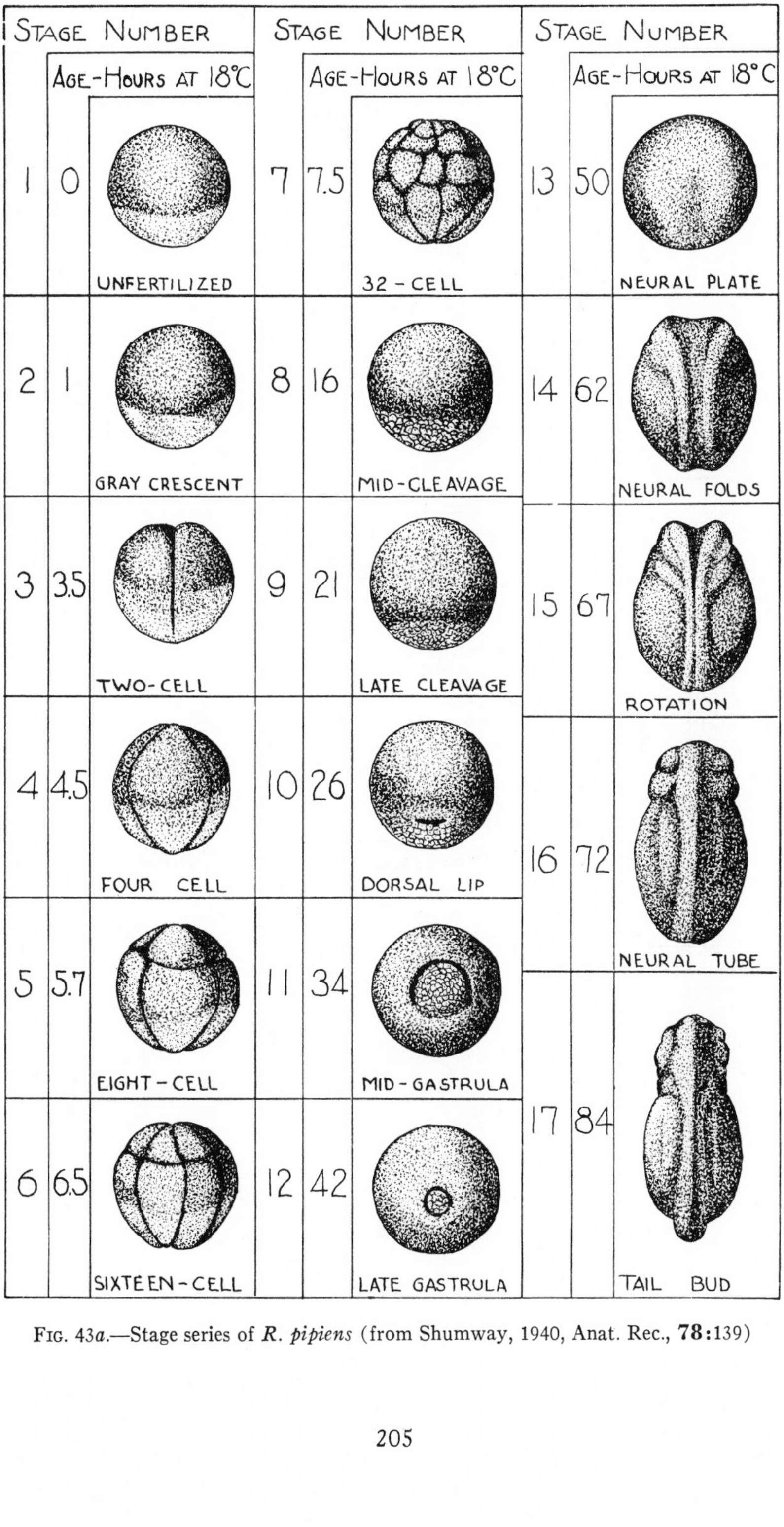

STAGE NUMBER	AGE-HOURS AT 18°C		STAGE NUMBER	AGE-HOURS AT 18°C		STAGE NUMBER	AGE-HOURS AT 18°C
1	0	UNFERTILIZED	7	7.5	32 – CELL	13	50	NEURAL PLATE
2	1	GRAY CRESCENT	8	16	MID-CLEAVAGE	14	62	NEURAL FOLDS
3	3.5	TWO-CELL	9	21	LATE CLEAVAGE	15	67	ROTATION
4	4.5	FOUR CELL	10	26	DORSAL LIP	16	72	NEURAL TUBE
5	5.7	EIGHT – CELL	11	34	MID – GASTRULA			
6	6.5	SIXTEEN – CELL	12	42	LATE GASTRULA	17	84	TAIL BUD

FIG. 43a.—Stage series of *R. pipiens* (from Shumway, 1940, Anat. Rec., **78**:139)

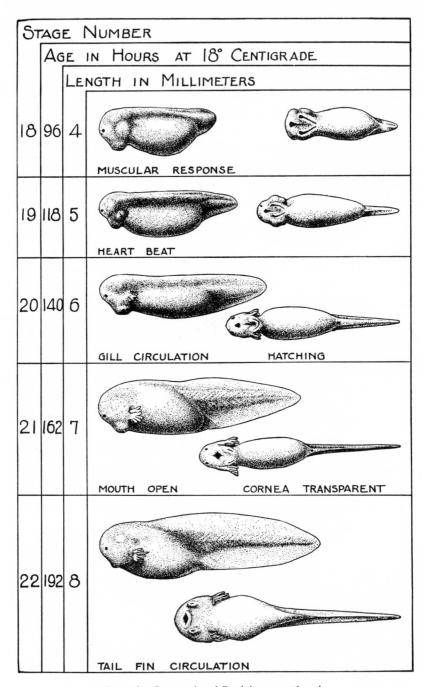

STAGE NUMBER			
	AGE IN HOURS AT 18° CENTIGRADE		
		LENGTH IN MILLIMETERS	
18	96	4	MUSCULAR RESPONSE
19	118	5	HEART BEAT
20	140	6	GILL CIRCULATION HATCHING
21	162	7	MOUTH OPEN CORNEA TRANSPARENT
22	192	8	TAIL FIN CIRCULATION

FIG. 43b.—Stage series of *R. pipiens—continued*

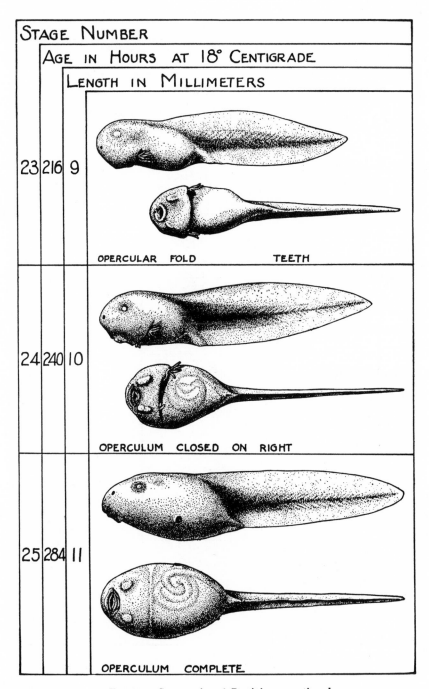

STAGE NUMBER			
	AGE IN HOURS AT 18° CENTIGRADE		
		LENGTH IN MILLIMETERS	
23	216	9	OPERCULAR FOLD TEETH
24	240	10	OPERCULUM CLOSED ON RIGHT
25	284	11	OPERCULUM COMPLETE

FIG. 43c.—Stage series of *R. pipiens*—*continued*

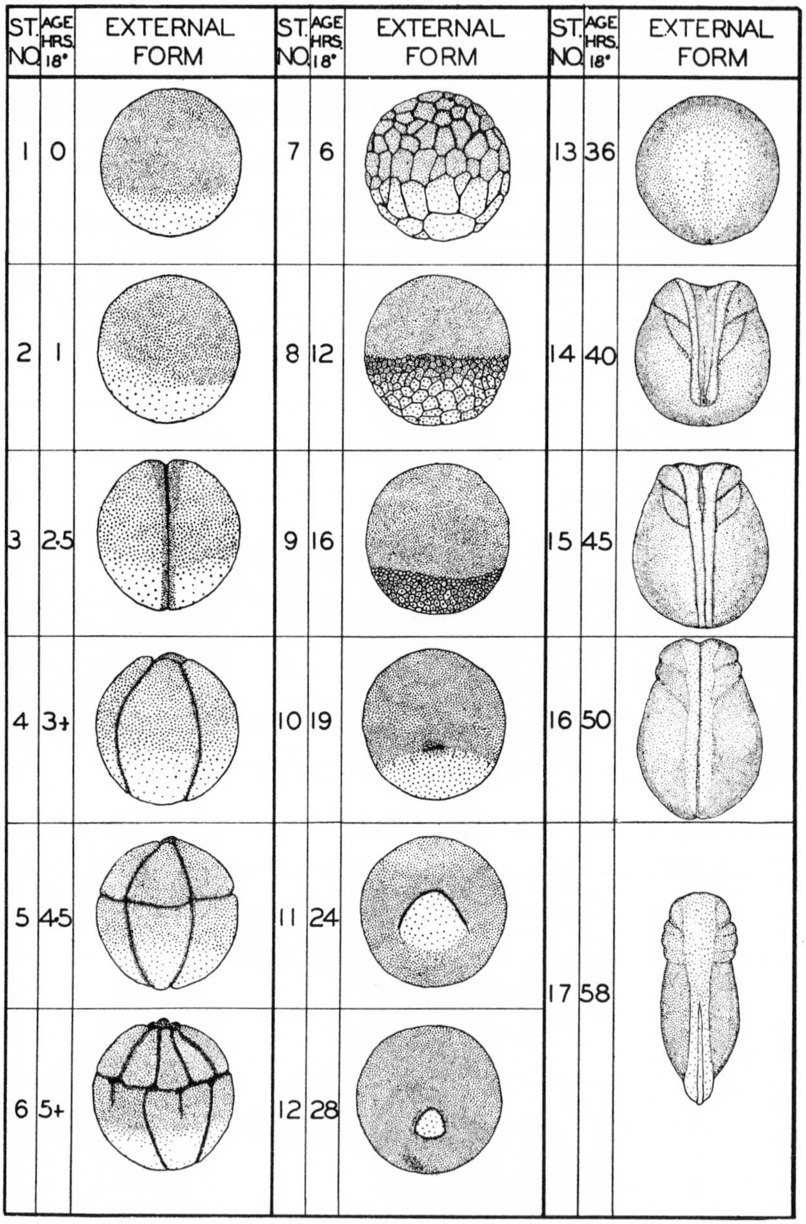

ST. NO	AGE HRS. 18°	EXTERNAL FORM	ST. NO	AGE HRS. 18°	EXTERNAL FORM	ST. NO	AGE HRS. 18°	EXTERNAL FORM
1	0		7	6		13	36	
2	1		8	12		14	40	
3	2.5		9	16		15	45	
4	3+		10	19		16	50	
5	4.5		11	24		17	58	
6	5+		12	28				

FIG. 44a.—Stage series of *R. sylvatica* (from Pollister and Moore, 1937, Anat. Rec., **68**:489)

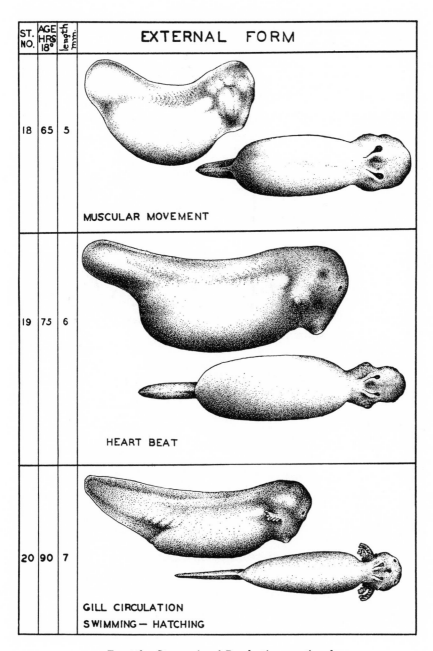

ST. NO.	AGE HRS 18°	length mm.	EXTERNAL FORM
18	65	5	MUSCULAR MOVEMENT
19	75	6	HEART BEAT
20	90	7	GILL CIRCULATION SWIMMING — HATCHING

FIG. 44b.—Stage series of *R. sylvatica—continued*

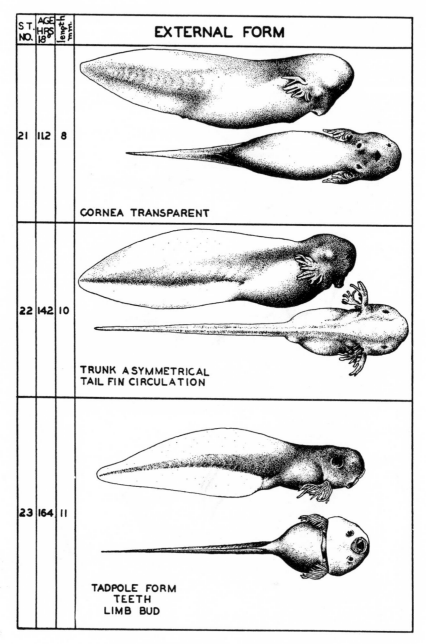

ST. NO.	AGE HRS 18°	length mm.	EXTERNAL FORM
21	112	8	CORNEA TRANSPARENT
22	142	10	TRUNK ASYMMETRICAL TAIL FIN CIRCULATION
23	164	11	TADPOLE FORM TEETH LIMB BUD

FIG. 44c.—Stage series of *R. sylvatica*—*continued*

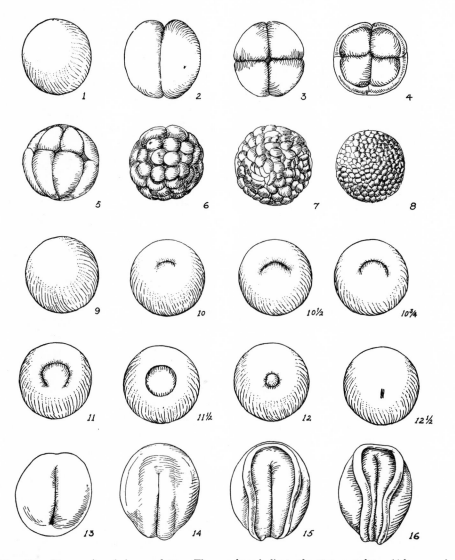

FIG. 45a.—Stage series of *A. maculatum*. The numbers indicate the stage numbers. (After unpublished photographs of Dr. R. G. Harrison, with permission of the author. Drawings by Miss S. E. Schweich.)

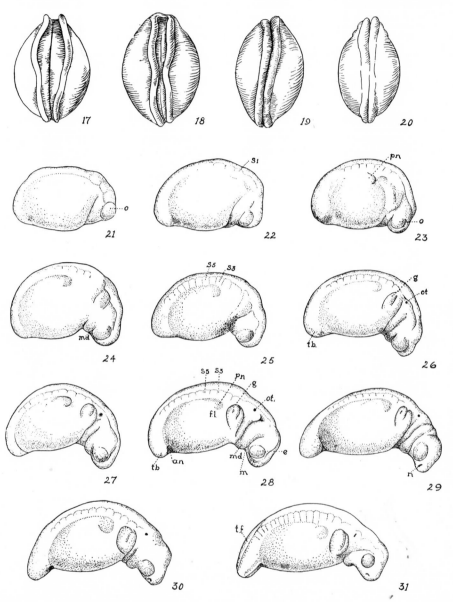

FIG. 45b.—Stage series of *A. maculatum*—*continued. an* = anus; *e* = eye; *fl* = forelimb; *g* = gills; *m* = mouth; *md* = mandibular arch; *n* = nose; *o* = optic vesicle; *ot* = otocyst; *pn* = pronephros; *s* = somites; *tb* = tail bud; *tf* = tail fin.

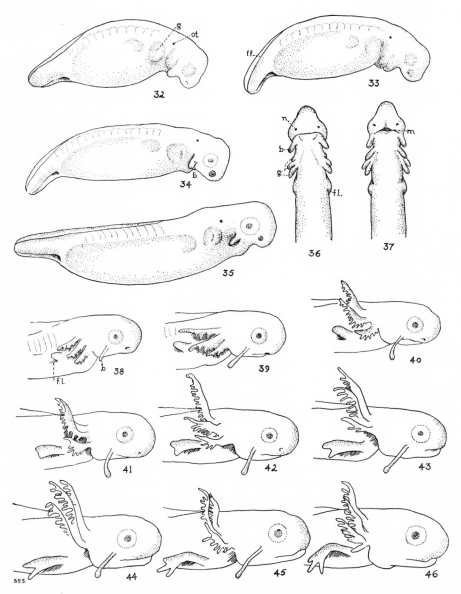

FIG. 45c.—Stage series of *A. maculatum—continued*. *b* = balancer; *fl* = forelimb; *g* = gills; *m* = mouth; *n* = nose; *ot* = otocyst; *tf* = tail fin.

INDEX

(A = Amphibians; C = Chick; P = Planarians; * = illustrated)

Acephalic monsters (P), 187, 188*

Adams, A. E., 133

Adelmann, H. B., 65, 108, 127

Agar
  bottom of dishes, 11
  dyed, for vital staining, 61

Alexander, L. E., 170

Alteration of cleavage plane (A), 75

Ambystoma, 16, 37, 62, 91, 96, 102, 112, 115, 116, 117, 119, 122, 135, 136, 139, 193, 194, 195, 198
  jeffersonianum, 86
  larvae
    feeding, 26 f.
    reflexes, 136 ff.
    regeneration, 192 ff.
  maculatum (punctatum), 16, 20, 37, 85, 86, 96, 109, 117, 122, 136, 138
    stage series, 20, 211*
  microstomum, 86
  opacum, 16, 22, 27, 85, 86
  punctatum; see *maculatum*
  tigrinum, 16, 21, 27, 86

Amphibian Ringer solution, 35

Anderson, P. L., 22

Androgenetic haploidy (A), 71

Androgenetic hybrids (A), 72

Animal pole (A), 58, 64

Anophthalmic heads (P), 187, 188*

Anterior duplications (A), 79; (P), 183,* 185

Antibiotics (A), 36

Anura (general), 18 f., 23 f.

Archenteron (A), 47, 48, 99

Archenteron roof (A), 48

Artificial insemination (A), 28 ff., 32, 34

Artificial parthenogenesis, 68 ff.

Atlas, M., 23

Axial gradients, 178, 179, 185, 187
  influence of, on head regeneration (P), 187

Axis determination in limbs (A), 93, 94*

Axolotl, 22, 23, 137

Bacon, R., 104

Balancer
  (A), 85
  determination of (A), 85
  transplantation of (A), 85, 87*
  vital staining of (A), 65, 66*

Ball tips, glass rods with, 5,* 8

Baltzer, F., 72

Basic procedures for operations (A), 41 ff.; (C), 147 ff.

Bataillon, E., 69

Beeswax, 12

Behavior pattern
  development of (A), 136 ff.
  stages (A), 137, 139

Beveridge, W. I. E., 160

Binocular dissecting microscope, 3

Bipolar regeneration (P), 183,* 185, 186

Bishop, S. C., 15, 37

Blastema
  in regeneration, 177, 178, 179, 183, 184, 192
  origin of (A), 178, 192, 193, 194

Blastocoele
  (A), 47
  implantation into (A), 120,* 121

Blastopore (A), 47, 48, 55, 63

Blount, R. T., 27

Born, G., 76

Braus, G., 90

Breeding habits (A), 15 ff.

Briggs, R., 27, 71, 72, 73, 76

Brondsted, H. V., 181

Bullfrog; see *Rana catesbeiana*

Burner, micro-, 4

Burns, R., 124

Butler, E. G., 194, 196

California newt; see *Taricha torosa*

Candling (C), 144, 148

Capillary pipettes, 4, 5*

Carbon marking (C), 154

Card, L., 143

Carpenter, E., 65

Cartilage stain
  after Lundvall, 146, 163
  after Van Wijhe, 163, 196

Casters, furniture, for raising of Amphibian embryos, 11, 12

Castle, W. A., 188

Check list of standard equipment (A), 44; (C), 145

Chick embryo, experiments, 143 ff.

Child, C. M., 127, 177, 178, 179, 181, 187, 188, 190, 191

Chloretone (narcotic), 40

Chorio-allantoic grafts
  (C), 153, 158 ff., 159*
  of eye primordia (C), 163
  of limb buds (C), 159,* 160 ff.
  method (C), 158, 159*
  of skin (C), 164

215

Chorio-allantoic membrane (C), 147, 158, 159,* 161

Cleavage plane, alteration of (A), 75

Coelomic grafts
  (C), 165, 169
  method (C), 165
  of limb buds (C), 165

Coghill, E. G., 136, 137, 139

Colcemide (teratogenic agent), 185

Coloboma (C), 170

Common newt; see *Diemictylus*

Competence, 114, 116, 117

Conant, R., 15

Concrescence, 58

Constriction of egg (A), 78, 81*

Convergence, in gastrulation (A), 55, 56, 58, 59; (C), 152, 153

Copenhaver, W. M., 103, 104, 105

Creaser, C. W., 29

Culture media (A), 34 ff., 43

Culturing methods
  for amphibian larvae, 26 f.
  for enchytrae, 26
  for planarians, 181

Cups, paraffined paper, 12

Curry, H. A., 73

Cyclopia (A), 109, 127; (P), 187, 188*

Dedifferentiation, 194, 197

Delayed posterior sections (P), 190

Demecolcine (teratogenic agent) (P), 185

Dempster, W. T., 20, 21

Determination, 83, 84, 101, 113, 177, 179

Detwiler, S. R., 28, 90, 102

Diemictylus viridescens, 17, 22, 33, 39, 62, 80, 91, 119, 122, 198, 200

Differential susceptibility, 126, 128, 134

Dinnean, F. L., 197, 200

Disease (A), 28

Dishes
  crystallizing, 11
  finger bowls, 11
  furniture casters for, 11, 12
  for operations (A), 11
  paraffined cups, 12
  Petri, 11
  Syracuse, 11

Dissecting microscope, 3

Distribution, range (A), 15 ff.

Dominance, physiological, 179

Dorsal lip of blastopore
  (A), 49, 51, 52,* 53,* 62
  transplantation of (A), 118 ff., 120*

Dossel, W. E., 10, 169

Driesch, H., 50, 75, 76, 78, 101

Duck embryo, stage series, 145

Dugesia (Planaria)
  anterior duplication, 179, 183,* 185
  bipolar forms, 183,* 185, 186

culture method, 181
delayed posterior sections, 190
dorotocephala, 181, 182, 186, 189, 190, 191
duplicitas cruciata, 183,* 186
experimental procedure, 181 ff.
head frequency, 187
head regeneration, 177, 183
lateral regeneration, 182, 183,* 184
oblique cuts, 182, 183,* 184
polarity, 178, 179
posterior duplication, 185
regeneration, 177, 181 ff.
tail regeneration, 177, 182
tigrina (maculata), 181, 182, 186
transverse cuts, 182, 183*

Duplications
  anterior (A), 79; (P), 179, 183,* 185
  by constriction (A), 78
  heart (A), 103, 104*
  limbs (A), 90, 194; (C), 160
  posterior (A), 80; (P), 185

Duplicitas cruciata (P) 183,* 186

Du Shane, G., 139, 171

Ear area, vital staining of (A), 65, 66*

Early reflexes (A), 136 ff.

Ectoderm, movements during gastrulation (A), 54,* 58

Edema (A), 28

Egg capsules
  (A), 16 ff.
  removal of (A), 37, 38*

Egg masses (A), 16 ff.

"Einsteck" method of implantation (A), 120,* 122

Ekman, G., 104, 105

Elongation, in gastrulation (A), 55; (C), 152, 157*

Enchytrae (white worms), 26

Endoderm formation (A), 57; (C), 150

Enucleation of egg (A), 74

Epiblast (C), 150, 154

Epiboly (A), 59

Epidermis, prospective (A), 59

Epigenetic theory, 75

Epimorphosis, 177

Equipment for operations
  on amphibians, 44
  on chick embryo, 143

Etkin, W., 133, 134

Exogastrulation (A), 127, 130 f., 131,* 132

Experimental ovulation (A), 28 ff.

Explantation (A), 97, 99*

Extirpation (A)
  balancer, 87*
  eye area in medullary plate, 107, 108,* 109, 110
  gill area, 97
  heart area, 106, 107
  lens epithelium, 116
  limb area, 101, 102
  optic vesicle, 111, 112,* 115

Illumination (microscope), 3, 73
Incubation (C), 143
Incubators, 143
"Individuation" (Coghill), 137
Induction
  by abnormal inductors (A), 122, 123
  embryonic (A), 113 ff., 118
  of lens (A), 113 ff.
  of neural tube (A), 113, 114, 118
  of secondary embryo (A), 118 ff., 120*
Inhibition of head formation (P), 187, 188*
Inner marginal zone (A), 56
Innervation, its role in development, 165
Insemination, artificial (A), 28 ff., 32, 34
Instruments
  glass, 3, 5*
  metal, 9, 5*
  sterilization of, 12
Invagination in gastrulation (A), 51; (C), 152
Inversion of axes, limb (A), 93, 94,* 95
Iridectomy scissors, 5,* 9, 92, 193, 195
Iris needle, 5,* 10, 146
Isolation experiments (A), 97, 99*

Jacobson, A. G., 115
Jull, M. A., 143

Kanatani, H., 185
Kaylor, C. T., 33
Keibel, F., 145
Knight, F. C. E., 22
Koecke, H., 145
Kollros, J., 86, 89
Kopsch, F., 15
Korschelt, E., 177, 181

Lallier, R., 128
Lamps, 3, 73
Landauer, W., 143
Late invagination (A), 55, 56
Lateral line placodes (A), vital staining of, 66*
Lateral regeneration (P), 183,* 184
Laterality, determination of, in limbs (A), 93, 94*
Lehmann, F. E., 127
Lens
  ectoderm, extirpation of (A), 116
  ectoderm, vital staining of (A), 65, 66*
  induction of (A), 113 ff.
  regeneration of (A), 197 ff., 199*
Leopard frog; see Rana pipiens
Liedke, K., 117
Lillie, F. R., 145, 158
Limb
  area, prospective (A), 90, 102
  axis determination of (A), 93, 94*
  chorio-allantoic grafts of (C), 159,* 160 ff.
  coelomic grafts of (C), 165
  duplications of (A), 90, 194; (C), 160
  extirpation of (A), 101, 102

flank grafts of (C), 166,* 169
regeneration of (A), 193 f., 195*
stages of (C), 145*
transplantation of (A), 89, 91*; (C), 166,* 169
Lithium experiments (A), 127 f.
Loeb, J., 69
Lundvall technique, cartilage stain, 146, 163
Lynn, W. G., 133

Malformations of head (A), 127; (P), 184, 186, 187, 188*
Manchot, E., 64, 107, 109
Mangold, H., 118
Mangold, O., 108, 111, 114
Maps of prospective areas (A), 50, 52*; (C), 151,* 152
Marbled salamander; see Ambystoma opacum
Marginal zone (A), 51, 56
Matthews, S. A., 40, 139
Medullary plate
  induction of (A), 113, 114, 118
  isolation of (A), 98, 99*
  prospective area of (A), 51, 54,* 58, 59, 64; (C), 152
  vital staining of (A), 54,* 64
Melanophores, origin (C), 171, 172
Membranes of eggs
  (A), 16 ff.
  removal of (A), 37, 38*
Mercurochrome (fungicide) (A), 28
Mesoderm
  formation of (A), 51, 62 ff.; (C), 150 ff.
  vital staining of (A), 54,* 62 ff., 63*; (C), 156, 157*
Metal instruments, 9
Metamorphic changes (A), 133, 136
Metamorphic climax (A), 133, 134
Metamorphosis (A), 26, 132 ff.
Metaplasia, 193, 194, 197
Microburner, 4
Microcephaly, 127
Micropipette (Spemann), 4, 5,* 146, 162
Microscope, binocular dissecting, 3
Miller, F. S., 185, 186
Monorhyny, 127
Moore, J. A., 20, 21, 22, 23, 24, 32, 72, 73
Morgan, T. H., 69, 177, 185
Morphallaxis, in regeneration (P), 177, 184
Morphogenetic fields (A), 100, 101, 104, 107, 108, 110, 111
Morphogenetic movements (A), 47 ff., 54*; (C), 150 ff., 151,* 152*
MS 222 (narcotic), 40
Murray, P. D. F., 160

Nakamura, O., 51
Narcosis
  (A), 40, 135
  reflex development in (A), 139

218

Nasal placode, prospective, vital staining of (A), 65, 66*
Needham, A. E., 177
Needles
  glass, 6
  steel, 10
  tungsten, 10
"Nests" for chicken egg, 146
Neural crest, transplantation of (C), 171 ff.
Neural tube, induction of (A), 113, 114
Neutral red, 60, 61, 154, 155
New, D. A. T., 149
Newman, H. H., 80
Newt
  California; see *Taricha torosa*
  spotted; see *Diemictylus viridescens*
Nicholas, J. S., 86, 90, 177, 194
Nieuwkoop, 24
Nile blue sulfate, 50, 61, 91, 119, 154, 155
Niu-Twitty solution (A), 35 f.
Noble, G. K., 15
Notochord, prospective (A), 51, 52, 55, 59, 63; (C), 152, 153, 154, 156, 157*

Oblique sections regeneration after (P), 183,* 184
Oliver, J. A., 15
Okada, Y., 22
Operation dishes (A), 11
  instruments, 3
  media (A), 34 ff.
Operations
  on amphibians, 61 ff., 192 ff.
  on chick embryos, 147 ff.
  general procedures for (A), 41; (C), 148
  on planarians, 181 ff.
Optic vesicle
  chorio-allantoic grafts of (C), 163
  extirpation of (A), 11, 112,* 115
  flank grafts of (C), 170 ff., 171*
  transplantation of (C), 170 ff., 171*
Organizer experiments (A), 118 ff., 120*
Orton, G., 15
Otocephaly, 127
Ovulation, induced (A), 28 ff.

Parabiosis (A), 123, 125*
Parmenter, C. L., 69
Parthenogenesis, artificial (A), 68 ff.
Pasteels, J., 51, 55, 56, 127, 154, 155
Petersen, H., 111
Physiological dominance, 179
Pickerel frog; see *Rana palustris*
Pipette
  capillary, 4
  micro (Spemann), 4, 5*
Pituitary injections (A), 28 ff., 30*
Planaria; see *Dugesia*
  anterior duplications of, 179, 183,* 185
  bipolar forms of, 183,* 185, 186
  culture method, 181

delayed posterior section of, 190
dorotocephala, 181, 182, 186, 189, 190, 191
duplicitas cruciata, 183,* 186
experimental procedure for, 181 ff.
head frequency of, 187
head regeneration of, 177, 182
lateral regeneration of, 182, 183,* 184
oblique cuts of, 182, 183,* 184
polarity of, 178, 179
posterior duplication of, 185
regeneration of, 177, 181 ff.
tail regeneration of, 177, 182
tigrina (maculata), 181, 182, 186, 190, 191
transverse cuts of, 182, 183*

Platinum wire loop, 7
Pleurodeles, 22
Plumage, pigmentation (C), 171 ff.
Polar heteromorphosis, 179, 183,* 185
Polarity
  limb (A), 93, 94*
  organizer (A), 118, 119
  Planaria (Dugesia), 178, 179
Porter, K., 72, 73
Prechordal plate (A), 48, 55
Preformation theory, 75, 76
Prenodal area
  (C), 150
  vital staining of (C), 157,* 158
Primitive streak
  (C), 150, 151,* 152*
  vital staining of (C), 155, 156, 157*
Prometamorphic period (A), 133, 134
Prospective organ-forming areas (A), 50 f., 52,* 53,* 54,* 61 ff.; (C), 150 ff., 151,* 157*
Prospective significance, 50, 83

Qualitative nuclear division, 76

Rana
  catesbeiana, 19, 115, 117
  esculenta, 114, 117
  palustris, 18, 24, 67, 111, 115, 116, 117
  pipiens, 18, 23, 29, 33, 69, 73, 77, 111, 115, 116, 117, 129, 135, 193
    stage series, 23, 205*
  sylvatica, 18, 67, 111, 115, 116, 117
    stage series, 23, 208*
  temporaria (fusca), 114
Range of distribution (A), 15 ff.
Rates of development (A), 20 ff.
Rawles, M., 147, 158, 171, 172
Rearing
  amphibian larvae, 26 ff.
  planarians, 181
Reconstitution, 177
Reflexes, origin of (A), 136 ff.
Regeneration, 176 ff.
  bipolar (P), 183,* 185
  blastema, 177, 192, 193, 194
  Dugesia (Planaria), 181 ff.
  field of, 178, 194
  of lens (A), 197 ff., 199*

Upper lip of blastopore (see dorsal lip)

Urodela
    general, 16 ff., 20 ff., 47 ff.
    regeneration of, 177, 192 ff.

Van Wijhe technique of cartilage stain, 163, 196

Viability
    of eggs (A), 32
    of sperm (A), 32

Vital staining
    of balancer area (A), 65
    of eye-forming area (A), 64
    of head structures, neurula (A), 65
    of Hensen's node (C), 156, 157*
    of lateral line placodes (A), 66*
    of medullary plate (A), 54,* 58, 64
    method (A), 49, 54,* 61, 63*; (C), 151, 154,
       157*
    of primitive streak (C), 156 f., 157*
    of prospective notochord (A), 54,* 55
    of prospective somites (A), 54,* 55
    of upper lip of blastopore (A), 62, 63*

Vogt, W., 47, 49, 50, 51, 56, 154

Waddington, C. H., 114, 152, 178
Watanabe, Y., 190, 191
Watch-glass technique (C), 147, 148
Watchmaker forceps, 5,* 9
Weismann, A., 76
Weiss, P., 76, 178, 194
Wetzel, R., 154, 155
White worms (*enchytrae*), 26
Willier, B. H., 158, 171, 172
Wilson, E. B., 69
Witschi, E., 124
Woerdeman, M. W., 64, 107
Wolff, G., 197
Wood frog; see *Rana sylvatica*
Wooden stand for instruments, 5,* 8
Wright, A. H., 15, 37

Xenoplastic transplantation, 96
Xenopus, 24

Yolk plug (A), 49, 56, 130

Zwilling, E., 160, 161